From Fat Boy to Fit Man

From Fat Boy to Fit Man

Eli Sapharti

A 'One-Step-At-A-Time' Story of Success

Jason Wood

From Fat Boy to Fit Man
Eli Sapharti
A 'One-Step-At-A-Time' Story of Success
Jason Wood

Disclaimer

your own choices, actions, and results.

This book is not a substitute for medical advice from board-certified medical professionals. Our readers should regularly consult with a physician in matters relating to his/her health, particularly with respect to any pre-existing health conditions.

Failure to obtain medical advice from your physician could be detrimental to your health. Results will dramatically vary from individual to individual. However, your health is paramount. Treat it with the highest respect as it is your most precious asset. Our goal is not to be a detriment but to promote healthy living – mind, body and soul.

We wish you all the very best in health and life.

From Fat Boy to Fit Man

Acknowledgement

When I squeezed into that airplane seat five years ago, I never imagined that that day would be such a pivotal point in my life. I never imagined that I would achieve so many personal goals. Heck, I didn't even know I HAD those personal goals. I most definitely didn't expect that I would make a difference in other people's lives. Nonetheless, here I am, healthier and happier than I even dreamed. Most importantly, I have found my life's passion in helping others help themselves. In turn, they are able to help others help themselves. And so on. It's a cycle worth continuing! The truth is by myself, I can only make a very small impact. I can only help that the branches rooted by my journey can form a collective by which to create impact that can be world-changing!

Throughout my journey, I have encountered hundreds

of people, who have, in one way or another helped me, encouraged me, or simply lent an ear whenever I needed it. It would be impossible to thank each of you individually. Yet to all of you, please accept my heartfelt THANK YOU!

Then there are those folks who have made a huge impact on my life and my success. They supported me, encouraged me, and believed in me even when I didn't believe in myself. I would like to take a moment to thank them individually.

First and foremost, I thank my dear mother, **Mireya**, for her unconditional love and for showing me by way of example how to be honest, loving, and kind, compassionate, patient, grateful and hopeful among many other positive attributes. **GRACIAS MIMA!**

There is no better way to experience unconditional love than one feels for their children. **Jessica, Moshe and Yehoshua (Shuy) Sapharti** are the reasons I live happily. They are the visions, who have carried me through the darkest moments of my life, and the vision who always makes me to want be the best I can be. You guys are my life! I love you!

A special thanks to **Maria Khawly**, who believed in me and my message, and actually pushed me to go out, spread the word, and make a difference. Maria, you have no idea how much your friendship, your help, your words of encouragement, and prodding have made all the difference in my world. THANK YOU!

Beginnings are sometimes the hardest. Not everyone is willing to give opportunity, but my dear friends: **Laura London** and **Adam Eckstein** gave me my first official shot at speaking publicly at *Laura's Fit & Fabulous Mom Contest*. Thank you, guys!

By myself, I am nothing, but collectively we can be great. This includes all my clients past and present. I would especially like to thank **Rick Wyckoff** and **Jennifer Babsky** for being amazing examples of what **One-Step-at-a-Time** can accomplish and for being true and loyal friends! Thank you!

I am a firm believer that "people come into our lives for a moment, a day or a lifetime. It matters not the time they spend with us, but how they impact our lives in that time." Thank you, **Cheryl, Madison, Jordyn** and **Tyler Hersch** for inviting me into your lives, if only for a moment.

I have been fortunate enough to have the opportunity to share my story, my message of hope, motivation, and inspiration with the masses. This has been possible because of the opportunities granted to me by some amazing media organizations such as *People Magazine, Good Morning America, Inside Edition, The Doctors, Huffington Post, AOL.com, Shapefit.com, BodyBuilding.com, DirectlyFitness.com, Natural Muscle Magazine, Competitor Magazine, Sun Sentinel, NBC 6, WPLG 10, America TeVe* among others. To you, I say THANK YOU!

Life is like a book. Some people are part of a page, others a chapter, and yet others the entire story. **Amy Henderson** is one *character* I hope remains with me until the very last word. Thank you for coming into my *story* and making it so wonderful!

Lastly, but definitely NOT least, **Mr. Jason Wood**! Sir, you are a gentleman and a scholar. When I was interviewing writers to co-author my book, I spoke to 'seasoned' and 'experienced' writers who dropped some big publishing names and talked a big game. Then I met you. You were humble yet confident, smart yet reserved, convincing yet subtle. Most of all, man, you were as passionate as I was about sharing my story. You believed we could help change peoples' lives. Ultimately, that was what was important to me. Thank you for putting my voice on paper. Thank you for the countless hours you spent going over these chapters and for your words of wisdom, encouragement, friendship and, even sometimes, tough love (God knows I needed some prodding some days). Without you, this book would not be a reality. You and I were meant to do this together. Thank you for everything!

This is just one more step of the journey I began in 2008. I look forward to continuing this journey together with you all **One Step at a Time!**

Eli Sapharti

Preface

Jason: OK, Eli, I have read a lot about you and I have watched your videos. You've made a massive transformation in your life. I see you reaching out to other people to pass on your secrets of success to them. The world wants to know: *How did you do it?* How did you get the weight off, keep it off and help others to do the same?

Eli: It's a process. The weight didn't come on in one day and it's not going to come off in one day either.

Jason: Here is my hypothetical question for you. I am 150 pounds overweight and I'm desperate to get in shape. How can you help me?

Eli: First of all, Jason, you're not 150 pounds overweight, and you've never been. You do not know what it feels like physically or psychologically. In order to understand the condition of being morbidly obese, you first need to understand and respect the struggle that I – and many others like me – have gone through being for lack of a better expression: HAVING TOO DAMN MUCH FAT!

Jason: I apologize. My goal is to understand what you have taught yourself and how it can be applied in order to help others.

Eli: That's fine. It's just very important to me that you understand what we have been through and what we go through as obese people.

Jason: But you're in fantastic shape. You're not obese at all. I just watched a video of you finishing a half-marathon.

Eli: Jason, understand something, the FIT person you see in front of you is only my exterior. Inside I still struggle with the FAT mentality that I know I will carry for the rest of my life.

Jason: Please explain.

Eli: After five years, I have come to the understanding that I am not fat. I know that I am physically in shape. That realization took me FIVE YEARS of being in shape to finally understand! Although I still struggle at times with the **Fat Mentality**, I have come to realize that I was never actually **FAT**. I was a person **WITH** fat.

Jason: OK, now you've thrown me off track. I don't understand. I thought you were fat?

Eli: No! I **WASN'T** fat. I **HAD** fat. Meaning, I had excess fat on my body in the shape of excess size and pounds. This fat used to define me. I was Eli, the wide-load; Eli,

14

fat ass; Eli, the bubble butt; Eli, *el gordo* and so on, labels people loved to call me. My size and my fat defined me. It named me. This weight convinced me that I was a number on a scale and a pant size in a department store. Nothing more.

Jason: I see.

Eli: After many years, I came to the realization that the weight I carried around with me was not ME. The excess fat did not and does not define me. Let me go one step further. Let me ask you a question.

Jason: Sure.

Eli: Am I fat?

Jason: Actually, you're in a lot better shape that I am. You are making me want to go to the gym.

Eli: So you would say that I am not fat then?

Jason: Not in the least.

Eli: Although I have lost over a hundred pounds and have maintained my weight, it took me almost three years really to understand that I was in shape. I kept telling myself that I was a fat guy who happened to lose a lot of weight. Literally, I had to retrain my brain to the reality that I am, in fact, FIT. To this day, I stand at the end of every 26K race in total amazement. I'm still surprised that I not only finished, but I actually ran my butt off for the whole race, all 13.1 miles.

Jason: Where did this quest to become FIT begin?

From Fat Boy to Fit Man

Eli Sapharti's
A 'One-Step-At-A-Time'
Story of Success

Jason Wood

Chapter One: The First Step

Eli: I worked for a company that exported consumer electronics. It was a job that required me to travel constantly. One evening I was in the airport in Miami on my way to Honduras for a sales call. Whenever I traveled, I always picked up a bottle of water before boarding the plane. This evening was no different. Well, actually, there was one thing different. I walked into a store, picked up water and headed to the cash register. A woman behind the counter tilted her head and seemingly looked me up and down. I didn't pay it any mind until she spoke to me.

"Good evening, will that be everything?"

"Yes, just the water. Thanks."

"That will be $2.69. Hey, you know something?" She asked.

"What's that," I replied.

"You know you're really good looking for a big guy."

"Ah...thank you?" I asked timidly.

"Oh, you know what I mean...I mean you are... well...I mean it's a compliment. Please don't take it the wrong way. I mean it in a good way."

I had already stopped listening. All I heard was: *DAMN, YOU'RE FAT! MY GOD, YOU'RE HUGE!* My thoughts drifted back and forth, my internal self-defeating negative banter winning out. And as I walked to the gate, all I heard was her voice repeating over and over just how fat I was. I replayed her comments forward and backward. I walked along realizing just how disgusted I was with myself. *"Eli, you are a fat piece of shit! You are nothing."*

I can still remember what I was wearing that evening: jeans, a long-sleeve shirt and a blazer. All of a sudden, I FELT my size. It was as if I never really understood just how big I was. I actually felt the fat jiggling through my body. I felt my blazer stretching tighter across my shoulders and my shirt sleeves cinching my arms. My jeans clung to my legs. My steps grew heavier. Every step I took seemed harder than the one before. It was as if 15 years of being obese had caught up with me in that one moment.

Jason: So, you never knew you were overweight before that moment?

Eli: Jason, it's not that I didn't know I was overweight before that day. Of course, I knew I was way overweight. That wasn't it. But that day, I finally cared. Can you understand that? I finally cared that I was so overweight. It really mattered to me. I guess you could say that I had a moment of clarity. It was an awakening. I became fully aware and cared about what had become of me!

Jason: So you had an epiphany?

Eli: And it didn't stop there.

Jason: So what happened next?

Eli: Well, my next mission was actually getting on the plane. It's easier than it sounds. You see, when you're a guy with my girth, a stroll down the aisle of an airplane isn't like a leisurely stroll through the park. I had to turn sideways so I wouldn't hit the seats on either side of the aisle. If I misjudged my trajectory, I would bang into other passengers getting settled which caused even further embarrassment. Once I reached my seat I had to lift the armrest and wedge myself into the seat. Then, the armrest had to be carefully lowered into the right position or my massive leg would press against the seat recline button forcing my seat backward, adding to my shame. I also had to be sure to move the seatbelt straps out of the way because once I sat down there would be no chance of reaching either strap beneath me. Then I would have to extend the seatbelt straps to their maximum length, suck in a deep breath, pull both ends of the seat belt toward each other and after a bit of wiggling and positioning, get the seatbelt fastened. At that moment, I could exhale and give an apologetic nod to the passengers on either side of me for my *get-in-the-seat-production*. I was just too embarrassed to ask for a seatbelt extension. (For those of you that don't know what a seatbelt extension is: it's a 24-inch extra seatbelt that clips into both sides of a normal seatbelt system. The extenders can be requested from a flight attendant or brought from home. Sold on the aftermarket in various colors, they are adjustable to accommodate more inches of girth).

For the duration of the flight, I rehashed the cashier's comments. The two hours I spent on that flight seemed more like a trial for a man in a capital murder case. The judge, jury, and prosecutor were convinced I was guilty of high crimes against myself. I'd tried to doze off, but my mind wouldn't allow it, circling around the facts. It was the longest two hours of my life.

When the plane landed in Honduras, I shuffled (sideways, of course) off the plane as quickly as I could, through customs and immigration, into a cab to my hotel. I needed a much-earned shower. The moment the water hit my body I began to regain my psyche. I told myself it was going to be okay. I just needed some rest. I closed my eyes for a few moments. And while steam filled my nostrils, that human feeling returned. *It must have been a bad daydream,* I told myself. *A good night's sleep and I'll be back to normal by morning.* Settled, I turned the shower off and opened the shower door.

My hotel was a business-class hotel. It was one of the perks of the job. The hotel's grounds featured pools, a breakfast buffet and a full-service office center. The room was well-appointed with a full sofa, a matching pair of barrel chairs, beautiful floral curtains and wall decorations. It had a desk, a mini-fridge and, unbeknownst to me, a massive full-length bathroom mirror directly facing the shower door and my naked body.

I stood motionless, frozen, staring at myself in the mirror. For the first time, in a long time, I looked at myself. I mean really looked at myself. Rolls draped my body in dramatic fashion. The sheer complete size of me was now on display. My weight and my size had taken over my life. It clicked. That was the moment. I knew in that very moment – standing there in all my obese glory – that I had reached a threshold. My thoughts bounced between airplane seat-belt extenders; sweaty trips up single flights of stairs; angry spoonfuls of ice cream; visits to *Big and Tall* stores; worn-out belts; gallons of soda; skin burns between my thighs; tiny toilet seats, accusing stares and smirks; bubble butt, *gordo*. It built and built, and before I knew it, I made a walk of shame to the bed. Something had to change. Something was going to change. I admitted to myself that it was out of control. I was out of control. My weight and this lifestyle were over. I didn't know what I was going to do, but I knew I was...

GOING TO DO SOMETHING!!!

"Faith is taking the first step even when you don't see the whole staircase."

Martin Luther King Jr.

STEP ONE:

DECIDE YOU WANT TO MAKE A CHANGE.

Before you can do ANYTHING, you must make a decision that you WANT to do SOMETHING. Notice that I didn't say NEED or HAVE, but WANT. This WANT must come from within YOU, not because others are doing it, or because your spouse, your kids, your friends or your parents are driving you crazy. In order for you to make the changes that last, you must WANT it for YOU! Period!!!!!!

Do you want to change? Forget about the HOW for now. DO you want to change? Are you willing to admit that you want to change? Do you want to change for YOU?

When you have answered YES to all four of these questions, you have completed STEP ONE!!!!

"The first step towards getting somewhere is to decide that you are not going to stay where you are."

John Pierpont Morgan

Chapter Two: The Second Step

Jason: So you had a breakthrough in the hotel bathroom?

Eli: I don't know if I would call it a breakthrough. It was more like the end of a very long road. I felt like it was a DUI checkpoint and I was way over the legal limit. I didn't know what I was going to do when I stood in front of the mirror exactly. I only knew that I really **wanted** to change.

Jason: So what happened next?

Eli: I got into bed, and tried to sleep. My mind wouldn't let me. I stayed up for hours, running through the day that began in a Miami store and ended in a hotel bathroom in Honduras. The current path of terrible health I was on had to come to an end. I wanted change. I decided I REALLY WANTED TO CHANGE. I went through the list of options I tried in the past:

1. Go on a diet? No! I tried every diet under the sun. The fad diets and short-term quick fixes left me worse off than when I started them. Most of the time, I actually gain more weight after the diet than before the diet began. Nothing worked for me in the past. Nothing!

2. Join a gym? For me, trying a gym always meant paying money, showing up one or two days then never going back. It never worked. Walking in to the gym always made me feel like I was the fat boy mannequin on display in a department store window. Seeing all the perfect bodies trying to lose five pounds compared to my fat ass with well over 100 pounds to lose? No, thank you.

3. Hire a trainer? A trainer would require that I embarrass myself in front of a professional AND the entire gym. That would be worse than joining a gym. Not for me. Not at all.

So with my options exhausted, I obsessed on the negative: my mind's default program of self-destruction. I already did the physical assault on my health. Now it was time for the psychological attacks to commence. The *Nevers* and the *Nots* came for a visit.

Jason: The Nevers and the Nots?

Eli: These are the voices that come when defeat is a far closer option than success. They always read from the same script. *"Eli, you are never gonna make it,"* says the Nevers. *"Eli, you're not good enough,"* says the Nots. Their lists include, but are not limited to:

- Maybe you're NOT meant to lose weight.
- You'll NEVER stick to this routine.
- You're NOT one of them. They're thin.
- You're NEVER gonna' be skinny. Why bother?
- You're NOT good enough.
- You've NEVER been good enough.
- You're NEVER gonna' make it.
- That life is NOT for you.

Jason: I guess it's pretty hard to make it when you aren't even in your own corner?

Eli: I wouldn't call it hard. I'd call it impossible.

Jason: But eventually you made it. How did you beat the odds?

Eli: After beating myself down, a light came on in my head. I came to the conclusion that I may NEVER have the body of a supermodel. I may NOT even make it all the way. But I was 100% sure that I WANTED and was WILLING to do something, anything.

I concluded that my approach would take the form of a two-part attack. I knew a major part of becoming healthy had to do with nutrition. It was clear that whatever was going into my body was a major contributor to my weight. Going on a diet, though, wasn't an option. I loved the food I ate; that would be a battle I'd surely lose. At that time, I ate just about everything under the sun. Pizza, cheese, sweets, bread, pasta, fats, food rich in sodium were all ingredients of my regular diet. I loved my food. I wasn't about to give up my food. Food was my comfort. Food was my security blanket. Food was my life. But what I COULD do was to cut out one single thing in my diet.

The first part was making a commitment. I COMMITTED to myself that no matter what else I did in my life I was COMMITTED to changing at least one thing I regularly put into my body. When the thought came into my mind, a small smile came across my face. Soda! At the time, I drank two liters of non-diet soda a day, every day. I COMMITTED to giving up non-diet soda. I said to myself no matter how long I lived and no matter what I had to do, I was COMMITTED to giving up the sugary sweet soda.

Jason: How hard was that for you to do?

Eli: Hard enough that even now when coaching a client, I recommend that if they believe they're unable to do it forever then try to start with seven days: A 7-Day commitment to giving up one thing from their diet.

Jason: And that's what you did? You committed for seven days?

Eli: No! I committed that no matter what, I was giving up soda for good. I gave it up. Don't get me wrong. I still ate the pizzas and fries and all the burgers, but I held my ground with soda.

You see, Jason, in order for me to make any progress I learned to build discipline within myself. Even the smallest **commitment** – when strictly adhered –builds discipline. **Discipline builds strength**. Strength carries you through all kinds of difficult situations. Before that conversation with myself, the scoreboard read: Eli 0 DISCIPLINE 100. After that conversation, the score changed: ELI 2 DISCIPLINE 98!!!! I was making up ground! I decided I WANTED to change, and I COMMITTED to give up one thing in my nutritional intake. For me, it was soda. For someone else, it might be ice cream or beer.

Jason: This was your second step?

Eli: Exactly! That was my second step!!

"All great change in America begins at the dinner table."

Ronald Reagan

STEP TWO:

COMMITMENT TO MAKING ONE SMALL CHANGE TO WHAT YOU PUT IN YOUR BODY.

Once you decide that you WANT to get healthier, start out by COMMITTING to make one small change to what you are eating daily and how you are eating. Follow through with this change for at least seven days. At the end of the seven days, repeat the COMMITMENT. This process will begin to build your discipline. Your DISCIPLINE is part of the key to your success. After completing three sets of seven days, you will have completed STEP TWO.

"If you're walking down the right path and you're willing to keep walking, eventually you'll make progress."

Barack Obama

Chapter Three: The Third Step

Eli: Two things happened while I laid in that hotel bed in Honduras. The **first** thing was a commitment to myself that no matter how hard it was, and no matter what it took I was going to give up one item from my normal daily diet. The **second** was a commitment to spend 15 minutes walking.

Jason: Why walking and why only 15 minutes?

Eli: As I lay in that bed, I decided I wanted to do some form of exercise that I could do when I was in town or out of town. I tried a spinning class in the past. After two minutes into the spinning class, I thought I was going to die. I didn't want to be in a gym with people looking at the FAT BOY trying to exercise. I didn't need the embarrassment. I wanted to succeed. I was committed to starting something that I knew I could finish. I figured 15 minutes wasn't long, and I was sure I could do it. Trust me, if I believed that I could only walk for 10 minutes, I would have chosen 10 instead of 15. I wanted to set goals that I KNEW I could achieve!!

With my **commitment** in place, I set out to put in my 15 minutes. Keep in mind, I gave up soda, but my pizzas, fries and burgers were more important to me than ever before. Nevertheless, I was embarking on a new challenge now.

With my shoes laced up and my best game face on, I headed out my door. I assumed that walking a mere 15 minutes would be a breeze. I assumed I could start walking, and before I knew it, my time would be up. I assumed too much!

After what felt like ten minutes, I looked down at my watch. Two minutes had passed. TWO MINUTES!!! I thought my watch had broken. How was that possible? Only two damn minutes? My breath was already picking up, and I could feel every step from the bottom of my feet to the hairs on the top of my head. All of my assumptions were wrong. Dead wrong!!

Let me try to describe the sensations in my legs. My shins ached. Shin splints couldn't begin to describe it. This was an ache deep in my muscles. It felt like a dinner fork scraping against my shinbones. Added to the shinbone-scraping was a burn and an itch that made me want to scratch my skin off!! I was now at the seven-minute mark. If I'd known it was going to feel like this, I may have never started!

Here I was half-walking, half-limping down the sidewalk, telling myself that I was halfway done. I told myself not to quit. Quitting wasn't an option. I pushed on. I committed and come hell or high water, I wasn't going to break my **commitment**!! I pushed on.

At long last, I finished. I felt as though I had run the *New York Marathon*. In reality, I had walked down the street then back for exactly 15 minutes!!

Jason: What happened? Why was it so hard? 15 minutes doesn't seem like it would make you fall apart like that. An hour maybe, but 15 minutes?

Eli: Imagine for a second that you're hiking.

Jason: OK

36

Eli: Now imagine hiking on sand with a 110-pound backpack on your back. Not only are you hiking on sand with a 110-pound backpack, but you have never hiked a day in your life. But wait! You aren't done yet. Add to the sand-hike and the 110-pound pack a ski parka, gloves, boots and a wool hat. Now, you would start to get the idea of what it felt like.

Before you even ask, I'm going to explain it to you. The ski jacket, gloves and hat represented extra fat on my body, creating a massive amount of heat. The backpack was the extra 110 pounds I carried. Ski boots in the sand was all that weight on my shins and feet while I walked down the sidewalk. The pressure from each step was a severe shock to my muscles, joints and tendons.

I didn't care if I was uncomfortable during my 15 minutes. I was pressing on no matter what. I committed, and I was going to see it through. I knew it would get better. I knew I would improve. At the very least, I would be able to tell myself that I was **DOING,** and not trying to do what I said I was going to **DO**. I knew then, and I know now that it is impossible to fail if you never give up. The failure comes from giving up, not from getting back up, dusting yourself off and going for it again!

I am a firm believer that **the word TRY is meaningless.** You either do something, or you don't do something. Saying that you will try is just another way of saying I don't think I can **DO!** I don't try to run a half-marathon. I run a half-marathon. I don't try to get up in the morning. I get up. I don't try to drive my car. I drive it! I may have needed to learn to drive, but that was only a matter of practicing **NOT** trying!! **Just forget the word try**

altogether!! Don't try to forget it. **Forget it!!** It's really that simple.

When I am in a coaching session with a client nowadays this is one of the first things that we address: Killing the word TRY. We are **doers** not triers. We are making commitments to ourselves. We are not trying to commit to ourselves. We already **tried** that. We have already TRIED diets, classes, fads, tricks, games and gadgets. They failed us. The trying failed us. That is why what I set out to do worked for me. I put away the trying. I started **DOING.** I started **COMMITTING. I started to build my internal discipline.**

Jason: So creating smaller steps built up your spirit?

Eli: Now you're starting to understand! You see I was so low that before I ever lost a single pound, inch or day of real physical progress, I first had to deal with my mind. I had to break the chains that I had put on myself. Trust me when I say that fat was just one of my many problems. It was just the external way for me to say to the world: *HEY!!! I'M NOT HAPPY WITH WHAT'S GOING ON THE INSIDE OF ME!!! I'M NOT HAPPY WITH MYSELF OR MY LIFE!!!*

Jason: Can you give me one example of the other issues you were battling with at the time?

Eli: Sure. In fact, I will give you two examples. I smoked two packs of cigarettes a day. I also suffered serious anxiety attacks for several years so much so that I only felt safe either at home or in a Target department store.

Jason: What the hell? In Target? You're joking.

38

Eli: I'm not joking. Not even in the least bit! A lot of people suffer from emotional issues, and I will devote some real time to talking about it later on. But I don't want to focus on those issues just yet. For now, let's stay focused on this step.

Jason: Step three?

Eli: Yes! Step Three!!

"The first and the best victory is to conquer self."

–Plato

STEP THREE

Now that you've made a change in your eating
habits, it is time to make a SMALL change in your
daily physical activities.

Most of you have probably been living a very
sedentary lifestyle or spent years not getting
enough daily physical activity. One problem many
people have when they decide to begin exercising in
order to lose weight is to TRY and go from '0-60' in
two seconds FLAT! Not only is your body unused to
such activities, neither is your MIND, which is the
most difficult to change. The human body is
resilient and is capable of MUCH more than you
think. It is the mind that is the toughest to break
and, therefore, is why you must 'train' it
slowly...ONE STEP AT A TIME!

One of the best exercises you can start with is
something that most of us can do easily...WALKING!
You don't need a gym membership, any special
machines, and you can't use the excuse that you
can't get 'there'.

Start out by walking 15 minutes every day. This will
not only help you get exercise, but most importantly
it will help you build commitment to your weight
loss journey.

"Patience, persistence and perspiration make an unbeatable combination for success."

Napoleon Hill

Chapter Four: Habits and Habitual Living

Eli: We all have habits. Some habits are healthy, and some are not so healthy. Nevertheless, we all have habits. In speaking with clients, friends and family alike, it never fails that someone approaches me with the question: *Eli, how can I BREAK this bad habit?* The habit might be smoking, drinking too much, or the obvious, overeating. My answer always brings a reaction of surprise. I tell them: *You can't.*

You see, I believe that you can't BREAK a habit. Whether good or bad, that habit is going to follow you around for life. Ask any recovering addict whether they ever find themselves thinking about the substance they stopped using. Ask them if they ever dream about it. In most cases, they will tell you: *of course,* they think about it. Most likely, they dramatically reduce the amount of time they spend thinking about it, but still...they think about it.

ELI: I REPLACE BAD HABITS rather than **try** to break them.

JASON: What does that really mean: replace bad habits?

Eli: It means that I replace poor eating habits with healthy habits. I replaced soda with water. I replaced smoking two packs of cigarettes a day with chewing gum whenever I feel the urge to smoke.

I identify the bad habit first. That is a key point. You have to know what you WANT to replace before you can replace it. Once the habit is identified, I can move toward finding its replacement.

Jason: So it's just as easy as replacing habits?

Eli: I didn't say it was easy. In fact, some say that quitting smoking is almost as hard as quitting heroin. No matter how hard you try, you will never be able to quit eating food. In many ways, food addictions can be much harder to overcome than drug addictions.

Jason: How so?

Eli: Without getting too deep into it now, I can say that food addictions are incredibly hard to overcome. Here's why...well, here's a few of the reasons why. Every store you go into has food for sale. Almost every airport, stadium, mall, school, street corner, gas station, work place, court house, casino, church or worship center, festival, social event or business center has food being offered for sale or given away for free. Even my bank offers free cookies!! There's no real escape from food. Every movie and TV show, and half the songs on the radio contain some food reference or another. The last time I checked they aren't offering crack cocaine in church or at the bank.

Jason: I didn't think about it like that.

Eli: And that is my second point about food addictions (or bad food habits). Few people take them seriously. So when you have the addiction, people just assume you love food. They offer you even more food. They say things like: *Give the big guy an extra serving. You know he can eat!* No one stops and says: **Wow! I bet that guy or girl may be really struggling with food. Maybe I should be polite and respectful to them. All of this might even be a lot of pressure on them.**

44

People can be very cruel to those with food addictions, or who have problems with overeating. I don't think there's a handbook on exactly how to approach an overweight person to offer them lo-cal food. Add to that, once you approach an overweight person with a lo-cal snack or meal, they most likely will not see your good intentions. All they hear is what I heard in the Miami Airport on my way to Honduras: *Hey, you're fat! You would be better looking and attractive if you weren't such a fat pig. Here, eat this lo-cal snack, piggy! So you don't further embarrass us with your fatness!!*

Jason: This topic is intense. I never really thought about it like that. I mean I try to understand what people are going through. Doing what I do for a living allows me to hear people's struggles and challenges, but I don't think I have ever interviewed a person about food addictions.

Eli: Think about it from another angle. Have you ever struggled with an addiction?

Jason: Of course.

Eli: What was/is the addiction?

Jason: I struggle with alcohol.

Eli: OK. So you're an alcoholic?

Jason: Wait a second! I didn't say I was an alcoholic. I said I struggled with drinking and alcohol. That's different.

Eli: Do you see how defensive you are right now? That's exactly how many overweight people feel when the topic of weight, dieting, exercise, fat, obesity, lo-cal foods, trainers, and so on comes up. It's uncomfortable, isn't it?

Jason: Point well taken.

Eli: The point wasn't to expose you, or to make you uncomfortable. The point illustrates that overweight people go through more than most can imagine. We're hooked on food, not something as 'glamorous' as booze or coke, so no one feels any sympathy for us. I'm sure if a drug addict joined NA, or an alcoholic joined AA, everyone would clap at the wonderful effort the addict made to improve his or her life. Food is different.

What makes the problem unique is the inability to hide the results of addiction or struggle. What I mean is this: With some breath mints and cologne, you might be able to mask a few extra drinks. How do you think an obese person is going to cover up an extra 100-200 pounds?

For the most part, if you tell people you join an overeaters' support group, you're going to hear clapping of a different kind. Most likely, you will hear clapping, followed by knee-slapping and loud laughter. People think it's a joke. They think overeating happens because we're fat lazy slobs. No one seems to realize that we can never quit food.

Drug addicts, at least, get the finality of quitting the substance that is killing them. If we quit eating, we will eventually starve to death. We have to eat. All of us have to eat. No one **has** to smoke crack or get drunk.

I am saying this not to diminish the great accomplishment in becoming clean or sober. Quite the opposite, in fact! I'm saying that **we overeaters** understand **you addicts** better than you might think. We have to take the recovery process to the next level, and because we still have to consume our addictive substance every day, we have to adapt. This is where the concept of replacing habits comes into play.

In the second step of my process, I gave up soda. I still needed to drink something. I couldn't just drink in the South Florida sunshine. At first, I replaced the soda with diet soda.

Jason: How big of a change was that for you?

Eli: It was about the same size change as going from beer to non-alcoholic beer.

Jason: Understood.

Eli: Soda was only the gateway though. Over time, my changes involved fats, carbs, sugar, dairy and on and on. One at a time, I addressed each bad habit and replaced it with something healthy. That was on the food side. On the fitness side, it involved a gradual staircase: walking 15 minutes back then to running half-marathons now. Things can change. **Things will change.** The key is to **replace** the bad with the good **One Step at a Time**.

This was the step that really started to turn my life around. Once I was able to replace the soda and keep my commitment to walking 15 minutes a day, I wanted to expand my progress. **Progress is exciting, but staying committed builds discipline.**

"Every day you may make progress. Every step may be fruitful. Yet there will stretch out before you an ever-lengthening, ever-ascending, ever-improving path. You know you will never get to the end of the journey. But this, so far from discouraging, only adds to the joy and glory of the climb."

Winston Churchill

YOUR NEXT GOAL

You already determined that you WANT change. You did that as a first step. Then you moved on to making one small change in your normal diet. That was the second step. After the diet-item change, you started exercising for 15 minutes a day. Every day! That was the third step.

Now you are building some strength and discipline. You should, by now, be able to see that you can put your mind to a goal and achieve it. The path that you are on isn't about the pounds on a scale. It isn't about what other people are saying, or aren't saying about you. This isn't about anyone but you. This is you doing you.

The next step is different. Now it's time to create a list: an honest list of five habits that you know are not good for you. It doesn't matter what they are. Put them on a list. You can list them in the spaces provided or anywhere you like. These bad habits may be either big or small. They may be food, alcohol, smoking, emotions, relationships, or any part of your life that you need to improve on. We aren't going to address those issues yet. Just writing them down is the goal and the fourth step. It's important to get those negative issues out in front, on paper and off your mind. Once you have them down, you have accomplished the fourth step.

BAD HABITS

1.

2.

3.

4.

5.

"Do the difficult things while they are easy and do the great things while they are small. A journey of a thousand miles must begin with a single step."

Lao Tzu

Break Down

At this stage of the journey, it's important to set the step process aside for a moment. I want to make sure that everyone is on the same page about overcoming the hurdles and challenges that come with facing new ground, or facing old ground in a new and different way. This is a **Break down.**

I understand the problems involved in making a major change. I understand the fears of failure. I get it. I've been there. I was *that guy* on the couch day after day, month after month, year after year. I was afraid. I was tired. I was sick of starting and stopping. That's all I did. I'd start something, but when it got too hard or I slipped up a little, I'd just stop. Every time I stopped, my self-esteem fell a little lower. Each time my self-esteem fell, it became harder to pick up that next diet or join that next gym or buy that next crazy fitness machine on a late-night TV infomercial. The Bottom Line: I WAS MORE AFRAID OF SUCCEEDING THAN I WAS OF FAILING!!!!!

Look, if you weren't afraid of succeeding, you wouldn't be reading this book. If this process was easy, everyone would've already done it. The whole world would be thin and perfect; none of us would ever have any problems, and we could all spend our afternoons sitting in a meadow throwing daisy petals at each other while drinking wheatgrass juice through a straw made from hay.

But that's not the case. This process is hard. We are not in a daisy-covered meadow drinking juice through a hay straw. Some of us are depressed. Some of us are experiencing some of the toughest times in our lives. We are hurting. We feel anger that we are in this position with no one to blame but ourselves. So now what?

Now, we have a little break down of sorts. Not the kind of break down that requires medication. No! Not the kind of break down that puts us on a 25-day diet of ice cream cake drowned in chocolate sauce. No! This is a different kind of break down.

I want to address a few things before going further. The first is simple enough: **we quit a lot.** We do!! We claim to have *tried* every diet under the sun, right? We claim to have joined gyms, bought machines, hired trainers, fasted, feasted and everything in between, right? And then we quit!? We quit. We stop doing whatever it was that we first started. We may have quit for millions of different perfectly good reasons. Nevertheless, in the end, we all quit.

WHY?
Why do we quit?

I believe one reason we often quit is due to our own image of ourselves. Do you like yourself? Do you like the way you look? Do you like the way you feel? Do you think you are a good person?

Take a few real minutes with me here. Understanding how you feel about yourself may be the most important thing you can understand in your life.

If you're like most of us, then you realized that you are not all you WANT to be. You may be overweight. You may have a host of other personal issues. No matter what the case is, we, humans, aren't perfect. We are in a constant state of change. We always have room for improvement. This book primarily deals with weight, fitness, health and well-being. However, these same rules, steps and guidelines can be applied to many different situations and issues.

Let's first put first things first.

HOW?

How do we solve big problems? How do we attack problems when they seem bigger than we are? So far in this book, we have outlined STEPS. Taking STEPS is an excellent technique to breaking down big, seemingly impossible-to-solve problems into smaller completely-solvable problems.

Do you know that mountaineers attempting to climb Mt. Everest stop at different base camps along the way? Each base camp offers a different level of support and respite from the daunting climb. If they climbed straight to the top of the highest mountain on earth, they wouldn't make it, most likely, perishing along the way. Now, mind you, these are some of the most experienced climbers in the world, yet they have a healthy appreciation for doing things in stages and steps. In fact, I'd go so far as to say their understanding of how important it is to take smaller steps along a journey toward accomplishing a much larger goal is what separates the pros from the novices.

On this journey, the process is much the same. You have a major goal you're working to accomplish. You have all the supplies you need, mental discipline, tools, and a guide. You know your direction, and you have a visual of what's at the top waiting for you. A NEW FIT YOU! Now, all you need to add to the list of supplies is a plan of stages and steps. Don't rush your climb. That's far too dangerous. Use caution in following the pathways that others who have been successful left behind for you to follow.

Starting with the simple **One-Step-at-a-Time** process that I developed allows you to progress gradually toward a new and healthier you. As you progress, you slowly start replacing your bad habits. At the same time, you inch forward in your exercise routine. Little by little, you build up your discipline. You will gain control in areas of your life that were once uncontrollable. None of us gained the weight overnight, so there's no reason to lose the weight overnight. The key to success is in the rebuilding. The rebuilding of you the way you want to be takes a little time.

Be patient with yourself! Of course, everyone's going to move at a different pace. Use the pace you can handle. Steady progress is better than shocking your system with a crash course in weight loss. Allow your body time to get used to the new routines you are carrying out. Rome wasn't built in a day, and you will not be totally transformed in a day.

Remember this is a process of learning how to care about you in a new way. Give yourself enough time to build. You are building a new you, a new way of looking at you. This is a pathway to success for a healthier future. This is why you are here. It is also the reason for this short Break Down. Now let's get back to work!!!

Together!!!!!!

"Everyone is a moon, and has a dark side which he never shows to anybody."

Mark Twain

Chapter Five: Target

Jason: Eli, in this chapter, I want you to tell me something about yourself that not many people know. I believe the more your readers know about you, the better. It's important that people reading your story know that you are more than half-marathons and healthy food. There's a real guy sitting in front me telling me about his life.

Eli: I'm actually glad you brought that up. I've wanted to talk about another aspect of my journey. This might be the perfect time to do so.

Several years ago, I was driving home from work. The day was no different from any other when out of the blue a strange feeling came over me. My chest began to tighten, and my breathing sped up. I tried to will it away, but that was no use. At first, I didn't know what was happening. Once I figured it out, it was almost too late. I put on my indicator and quickly pulled the car off the freeway. Gasping for air, I dialed 911. The operator tried to calm me, but it was no use. I was already going off the deep end.

It didn't take long for the ambulance to arrive. I was whisked on to a gurney and straight into the ambulance. As soon as I told them about massive chest pains, sweats, trembling and shortness of breath I was put on an IV, given beta-blockers, and hooked up to a heart monitor. We raced to the nearest hospital where I was rushed in. My shirt had already been peeled away to allow the technicians to perform the EKG, and a series of other tests. At last, the ER doctor came in.

"Doctor, I know I'm having a heart attack. Please allow me to call my wife and tell her. Please let me call her. I know I'm dying."

The doctor looked at me with a half smile and gently shook his head. "Eli, you aren't dying. You aren't having a heart attack. What you are experiencing is a panic attack."

Jason: A panic attack?

Eli: Yes, an extreme panic attack. I used to suffer from horrible panic attacks. I don't talk about it a lot, but I suffered and often.

Jason: Wow!

Eli: The doctor explained that a panic (or anxiety) attack can feel exactly like a heart attack. The fears and discomfort cause a flood of adrenaline into the system. The body goes into shock. It thinks something is dramatically wrong and reacts with a fight-or-flight response. Even though, there really isn't anything wrong and there is no need to sprint away or fight a tiger; all that adrenaline and energy freaks out the person experiencing it. The heart races, the chest and muscles tighten, you sweat, breathing gets heavy, and you mentally and physically gear up for the fight of your life.

Jason: And you were just driving down the road?

Eli: Exactly! That's why it's called a panic ATTACK! It comes out of nowhere and grabs you wherever you are and whatever you are doing. No warning. Physically, I was in my car driving the same freeway I always drive. Mentally – and emotionally – I might have been fighting a bull in an arena or jumping out of an airplane. My body responded to what my mind told it rather than what my eyes saw and my ears heard. It was a massive overload to my system.

The doctor recommended I see a psychiatrist. I booked an appointment at once. I was more than willing to try anything to make the anxiety go away. The psychiatrist was nice enough and after a series of questions and an examination prescribed some drugs to ease my anxiety and get me back to normal.

Jason: Did that help? I mean did the medication ease your mind?

Eli: Actually, at first, the medication had the reverse effect. I started to feel suicidal.

Jason: Yikes!

Eli: Medication can be hit or miss. Everyone's different. Medication can produce a different reaction in each person taking it. The medication I first received was most definitely a miss. The panic and anxiety actually increased. It was pretty clear that meds alone was not going to be the solution. I was referred to a psychologist for additional counseling.

Jason: What's the difference between a psychiatrist and a psychologist?

Eli: Simply, the difference is that a psychiatrist is a medical doctor while a psychologist is generally a PhD.

Both can treat mental disorders, but only a psychiatrist can prescribe medication or perform medical procedures.

Jason: So what did the psychologist do?

Eli: We started by talking about what my life was like, how I went about my daily business. I did most of the talking; he did most of the listening. In the first few sessions, we went over a lot of the basics of my life. I described how anxiety would sneak up on me without warning and leave me paralyzed. He had me walk him through a typical day. Through this exercise, I started to realize that the anxiety I felt was no small part of my life. It was as much a part of my life as breathing or putting my clothes on in the morning.

Jason: Will you share another example of how anxiety and panic attacks affected your life?

Eli: I can give you a zillion examples. For one, I always had to take the same route to work in the morning and back home in the evening. When I say the same route I mean using the exact same lanes, turning at exactly the same place every day. To make even the slightest variation would cause my mind to go into panic mode.

I would go to work and return home. Other than at those two places, I felt totally out of place. I did not enjoy going out to eat, spending time in the park with the kids, or catching a ball game on the weekend. There was only one other place I felt comfortable going.

Jason: And where was that?

Eli: Target.

Jason: What the hell? Target? Why Target of all places?

Eli: I don't really know. Maybe it was the well-lit spacious aisles. Maybe it was the fact that everything was in there. I mean you had a Starbucks at the front of the store, CDs in the back of the store. Everything a person needed was right there in the store. I could walk the aisles with the wife and kids, or just by myself. Every weekend, we went. Like clockwork, we would arrive, park, get the over-sized grocery cart and stroll around Target. What can I say? The store gave me peace of mind.

Jason: Well, I can say I've gone into Target for a single toothbrush and three hours later left with food, CDs, socks, a PlayStation, bicycle tires, fishing gear and 20 other items I didn't know I needed until I went in that damn store.

Eli: That's just it. I got the feeling that everything was okay because anything and everything was there. I knew what was located on what shelf. There was no guesswork. There was no mystery to it. Few things changed. It was a controlled environment. Even the temperature was predictable. I felt great comfort in Target and rarely suffered any kind of attack in the store.

Jason: Who would have thought? Actually, it makes sense to me. If your fears were based on unpredictable events or what-ifs, then I suppose doing the most routine tasks could bring you peace and keep you calm. It was as if by shopping and choosing the things you

63

knew would be there waiting for you gave you some sense of control and power over your situation.

Eli: It did. It was routine and while shopping, a comfort zone where I was totally able to maintain. Trust me not every place gave me the peace I found in Target.

I never liked being in public. For me, traveling was an absolute nightmare. I wanted to avoid traveling at all costs. However, this was nearly impossible because of my job. I was constantly traveling. Each trip was another chance to have a panic attack. My greatest fear was passing out. I was afraid of having an attack in an airport somewhere, or in some foreign country and passing out. You see, when the attack comes you believe that you're going down. Lights out! Out cold!

Jason: How did you deal with that? What did the psychologist tell you to do?

Eli: He told me to go ahead and pass out if I needed to pass out.

Jason: Your psychologist told you what!

Eli: Yep. He said, *"Eli, if you think you're going to pass out just relax and go ahead and pass out. See what happens."*

Jason: Did you stop seeing this psychologist?

Eli: Actually, I took his advice on my next trip. I was seated in the airport when the attack began. All of a sudden, the symptoms rushed in. I started sweating and breathing heavily. I looked around for someone to help me if I did actually pass out. Everyone appeared busy and uninterested in my state of being. Yet I could feel this surge of fear climbing up the back of my neck and at the same time, into my chest. There it was: the unforgettable feeling that I was going to pass out. I was in a panic. Then I remembered my psychologist's words: *Eli, if you feel like you're going to pass out, then just let yourself pass out. The more you resist the more it will persist.* I didn't know what else to do so I told myself: *The hell with it, Eli, just go for it... pass out!*

Jason: Did you?

Eli: The strange thing is no, I didn't pass out. I started to black out and even leaned off my chair, but the moment I stopped fighting the feeling I lost the urge to pass out. It was like the fear of passing out was what was making me go blank. Realizing there was absolutely nothing I could do about it actually woke me up. Admitting that I was powerless gave me power.

As time passed, I began to gain more confidence in my ability to maintain. I kept seeing my psychologist while my psychiatrist found the right medication to work with my system and reduce my anxiety level.

The thing to take from this is that when I needed help, I gave in and asked for help. Everyone likes to think they can manage all of their problems by themselves, but that doesn't always work. Sometimes the problems we face are too big to handle alone. Talking helps. Seeking professional help can work. Pride doesn't work. Having too much pride, believing you can do everything in life alone can be dangerous. I believe it's important to use the tools that are out there to help you help yourself. I would never suggest implementing the techniques in this book without first speaking with a physician. We can all leave the hero act for characters on TV. But if you insist on being a hero, be the kind of hero who knows when to call for back up.

Through the process of overcoming my fears, I was able to solidify the process of breaking down things into steps. When I gained ground on my issues, I built confidence and strength. Of course, I had relapses. Of course, I struggled, but I never quit. I always pushed on. With the help of people around me, I learned how to live again. Remember major change normally doesn't happen in one day. It takes time. We all have some time. We have time to build. Building internal strength is the key to building lasting success. It isn't about becoming a model or movie star. It's about becoming the person you like. It's about looking in the mirror and being proud of you. Not the kind of pride that gets you in trouble, but the kind of pride that comes from respect of your journey. The journey we all are on, to be the best people we can be. That, for me, is what it's all about.

"We delight in
the beauty of
the butterfly,
but rarely admit
the changes it
has gone
through to
achieve that
beauty."

Maya Angelou

Moving Forward From Here

Change happens in life. Change can be scary. Change is the unknown approaching us whether we like it or not. Change does not care if we're ready, or made the proper arrangements. It just comes. I believe the key to change is allowing it, welcoming it and embracing it with open arms.

There have been times in my life when I really needed help. The last chapter was a perfect example. I was a mess. I was down. I wasn't able to continue living the way I had been. **So what did I do about it?** That's obvious: **I got some help!! I asked for help.** I know that is a major issue for some.

Asking for help can be one of the scariest experiences of one's life. However, it is key to overcoming problems that are too large to solve alone. There's nothing wrong with asking for help. Let me say that again. There is nothing wrong with asking for help! And one more time for those stubborn few, like me, who need to hear something three times before it starts to sink in. **THERE IS NOTHING WRONG WITH ASKING FOR HELP!!!!**

Depression, anxiety, mood and mental disorders are serious things. They are not to be taken lightly. Yes, of course, it's not glamorous to walk into a doctor's office and tell the nurse you're there for some emotional or mental condition. Your friends might not understand. Your spouse might tell you that all you need is a hot bath and a day off. Let me say it again: If you feel the need to see a professional about your emotional or mental state, do so. Do not wait another hour of torturing yourself and your loved ones. Forget pride and embarrassment and **ask for help**.

Your mind is the most valuable thing that you have. In fact, it's one of the few things you have. Your house, car, valuables and earthly comforts can disappear in the blink of an eye. Even your loved ones can be taken from you, but your mind will be 100% with you for the rest of your life. I strongly suggest you take good care of it.

Taking this walk of self-improvement will be very difficult at times. The world can be cruel. Be kind to yourself. Allow yourself the best chances of success by enlisting excellent team members. A physician should be involved with any weight-loss programs you begin. Never rush out and start an impulse crash diet/exercise program without first consulting with your doctor. That covers the body, but what about the mind?

Mental health is just as important as physical health; sometimes even more important. You can have six-pack abs and still want to jump off the nearest bridge. So it's essential to listen to yourself. Never let pride or embarrassment push you around. Get professional help if you have any question about your mental state. You want to be healthy in mind, body and spirit.

Now let's get back to the task at hand...
Getting healthy!!!

"The will to win, the desire to succeed, the urge to reach your full potential...these are the keys that will unlock the door to personal excellence."

Confucius

Chapter Six: Pen and Ink

Jason: The last few chapters about your struggles have been pretty revealing. How can your personal challenges best help others?

Eli: It's crucial for readers to understand fully that they are not alone in their struggles with **themselves**. I have been there. I know. I know them. I know what they struggle with. I believe that **90%** of the people reading this book haven't started **Step One** yet. I know I would've told myself that I'd start the steps as soon as I finished the book. Of course, once I finished, the book would've gone straight on my bookshelf, right beside the stack of other books I'd read on health and weight loss and never opened again.

Jason: So how is any real progress going to be made if your readers don't start the work?

Eli: It **can't** and it **won't**. The progress **won't** start until people realize that the time to take action is **now**. I mean **RIGHT NOW!**

If you're one of the 90% who haven't started **Step One, Two** and **Three,** you need to **STOP!**
STOP reading any further than this chapter.
STOP making excuses about why you haven't started taking action.
STOP doing anything else and listen to me for a minute.

Special moments in life can change things for you forever. These are the moments you'll look back on years later and say to yourself: *That was the day I changed. That was the day I knew I would never be the same.*

I want this to be that day for you. I want this to be the day you promise yourself that you had enough; you want more from your life and you are committed to finally doing something real about it. **YOU** have control. **YOU** are the only person who can make this decision for yourself. It's time. There is no better time than right now to make the **Decision**. Make the **Decision** and go for it.

I want **YOU** to experience the overwhelming joy of waking up every day a little bit healthier than the day before. I want **YOU** to gain all the energy that is waiting for you, inside you. I want **YOU** to look in the mirror and see the pounds melting away. I want **YOU** to know what I already know. **YOU** can do this. **YOU** have everything you need to win inside you. I want **YOU** to walk down the street excited to pass a store window, excited to see your own reflection in the glass. I want **YOU** to be free.

Yes, there's work to do. Let's get started on that work right this minute. I want you to make a commitment to yourself right now, right here in this book. Go get a pen (not a pencil). The next page contains a simple contract I want you to sign with yourself.

YES! I'm serious. Get the pen. While you at it, open your mind up a little.

I_____ do hereby agree to
begin the first three steps in this book. I agree to move forward with following commitments to myself.

From this day forward, I do hereby agree to commit to walk/exercise for exactly_____ minutes a day, every day.

From this day forward, I do hereby agree to commit to remove _____
(food item to be removed)
from my daily calorie intake. If I feel the need to replace it, I will replace it with the healthy alternative of

_____.

From this day forward, I promise to remember:

I am worth investing in.
I am worth believing in.
I am worth struggling for.
I am worth giving up my guilt

From this day forward, I promise to:

Understand I have started.
Understand I have already progressed.
Understand I have succeeded and I will continue to succeed.

I understand I have now taken a different path in my life. I understand and agree that quitting is not an option because I am in control of my choices, life, and my rules.

Signed _____date / /

73

Congratulations!!!

Now you have put pen to paper to make an agreement with yourself. You will not break your agreement with yourself because you are making the rules and the decisions. You are going to build your inner strength and confidence. You are going to learn to crawl, to walk and to run. I will be there with you for support, but this is a journey that you are taking for you. This journey is not for your children, spouse, boyfriend or girlfriend. This journey is not for your job, your friends or anyone you want to impress. This journey is for you and you alone.

TIPS: Exercise

When choosing the amount of exercise you're going to perform each day (including today), choose an amount of time you're sure you can accomplish for the next seven days. Do not set a goal that you'll start today and end up bailing out three days from now. I started with 15 minutes. You've already read about how I itched and burned like my body was on fire. If you need to start with five minutes, start with five minutes. It doesn't matter the amount. What matters is that you choose to stick to that time. If it's five minutes and you finish those five minutes, you're done for the day. Do not put in an extra five or ten minutes because you feel great. Stop at five! Stick to your agreement. Don't do more; don't do less. You are building inner discipline and self-control. *'Slow and steady wins the race.'* If you do too much in one day, you may not be able to maintain that pace all week. Then your new schedule will get out of whack. Stick to your signed agreement. Aim low not high when you first get started. This is not the time to challenge yourself beyond what your signed agreement states. The key is to start and to stick with it. The real challenge will not be the short amount of time you spend exercising. The real challenge will be sticking to the agreement over the long haul.

TIPS: Food

We all know when it comes to food the real battle begins. Food is our comfort. At times, food is our best friend. At other times, food is our worst enemy. Food, food, food, what are we going do about food? It can be such a personal topic, but like it or not that is why we are here. Food is the reason I wrote the book. Food is the reason you're reading the book. We have to get control of the food we put into our bodies. Just like you,

75

I've cried over food. I have lied over food. I have eaten a whole tub of ice cream with mad vengeance. I have eaten cake angrily. Like you, I have done it all. And now we are here together. We are here to, once and for all, show food who's the real boss.

When choosing a food item to remove or replace, do so carefully. If you toss out your favorite food first, you are surely going to feel the pain. I suggest picking a daily food item that you know is contributing to your fat. Choose a food item you know you can –and should live – without. If it's a double cheeseburger and you aren't ready to give it up, then don't choose the double cheeseburger. If you live for fries, enjoy those fries for just a little while longer.

I chose soda. The amount of soda I drank and the amount of sugar I consumed every day was incredible. I did not give it up; I replaced it. I traded it for diet soda. That was it. That was my dietary change. It was my first step. I don't want to tell you what food item to give up and what food item to keep. I **DO** want to tell you that once you signed that agreement, you agreed to give up your guilt. So please don't feel guilty giving up bacon (for example) and continuing to eat steak. That is just fine. The goal is not a massive overnight transformation. In fact, the opposite is actually true. This, by design, is a slow and steady transformation of you gaining some control over yourself and what you **CHOOSE** to eat and what you **CHOOSE** not to eat. If you need to, go easy on yourself at first. Choose a food item that isn't too difficult to replace or give up altogether. We can get to the tougher food items later. There will be time for that.

Do not play tricks with yourself. For example: If you don't eat pie, ice cream and brownies, then don't add them to your food routine. Stick with your current diet, but make changes based on your current diet.

Use your head when replacing food. For example: Replacing a double cheeseburger with a double pork burger with cheese is not going to work in this program. You know what is good for you and what isn't. You know exactly what I'm talking about because you and I have already tried a thousand diets which we eventually (after a few hours) cheated on. This is not a diet. Say it out loud! **THIS IS NOT A DIET!!!!!** This **IS** learning how to retrain your brain to build your self-control, self confidence and your ability to choose food rather than food choosing you.

I believe in you. I am speaking to you. I wrote this book for you and I know that you can do it. These are not just words. This is something I have already done. It worked. I changed. I made it, and I want to help you make it. Together we can do it **One Step at a Time** until you're doing it all by yourself. Getting in shape was the single greatest gift I have ever given myself. It changed my life so much so that it compelled me to tell you that it is, in fact, possible. You can achieve your goals.

Thank you for this opportunity! –Eli

"Those who are happiest are those who do the most for others."

Booker T. Washington

Chapter Seven: Tools For Battle

Of the many terms used to describe the rollercoaster of weight loss and fitness, I've heard (and used) 'struggle,' 'battle,' 'fight,' and 'war,' just to name a few. If this journey is a battle in your mind, then it's a battle I want to help you win. Like any other battle, you're going to need as many weapons (or tools) as possible to win it and, ultimately, to win the war.

The war itself is not you against food. It is not you against a pair of jogging shoes, the track or even the scale. Those are all just pawns of war. The real war being fought is within **YOU**! The key to victory lies within the truth and the ability to be honest with yourself. You want to succeed. You want to win. You want to get healthy. You want to look in the mirror and smile at the person looking back at you. I know this. I looked in the mirror in that Central American hotel bathroom, and did not like what I saw. I knew I had to start by making, at least, one commitment that I was sure I could keep with myself. I actually made two. The first, as you know, was removing or replacing one unhealthy nutrition choice. For me, it was soda. The second choice was walking for 15 minutes a day.

I'm often asked: *Eli, 15 minutes? Really? That's all it took? You made this total transformation just by walking for 15 minutes a day?* The answer is simple: NO! No, I didn't lose all the weight and start running half-marathons by walking for 15 minutes a day. What I **DID** do by walking for 15 minutes a day was begin to retrain my brain. I began to arm myself with some tools. The first tool was **accomplishment.** I set a goal, and I accomplished it. The feeling of accomplishment was

79

refreshing and added a tiny inch to my confidence. I thought to myself: *Well, if I can accomplish this one small goal, maybe I can accomplish another small goal.* And so on and so on until accomplishing goals no longer scared or intimidated me. I started to believe in my ability to set out and **FINISH** what I started.

I want to arm you with some of the tools that will assist you in your journey. Keep in mind we are fighting not only with fat and weight, but also the mentality that comes along with it. These tips will help keep you in a focused mindset of accomplishing small goals. There are no steps backward. There is nothing to fail. **YOU** are setting up the rules for **YOU**. I am only providing a few tips and cheering you on along the way. Some of the tips may sound silly or oversimplified. However, I can tell you from my own experiences that they help keep your mind sharp and focused on winning the war rather than giving all your power to the enemy called: *I can't; I'll try; I'll do it later; I wish I had her body; I wish I looked like him and so on.*

One

In years passed, I *cleaned the plate* when eating dinner. No matter how large the serving, I made damn sure it was all gone before I got up from the table. I don't know if I was programmed from a young age, or just adopted the habit along the way, but when they served it, I ate it All!!! I was the worst offender at dinnertime. Countless calories were consumed. I took in **far** too many calories to burn off sleeping. One evening after beginning the **One-Step-at-a-Time** process, I realized that no one was forcing me to eat every bite off my plate. I had my own free will. I could choose to do whatever I wanted to with my dinner. So I tried an experiment. I ordered a normal

80

dinner, but I asked the waiter if he would box up half of the meal before he served me. **YES!** Yes, you can do that. It's not a big deal. I didn't care what anyone thought about it. I cared only about what **I** thought about it. It's **MY** dinner, and it's **MY** body, right? I ordered what I was hungry for, and an interesting thing happened that night. I felt totally comfortable eating all that was on my plate. I was relaxed. I didn't feel like a pig or that I was gorging myself. I simply ate dinner. By the time I finished, I felt full. I didn't need that second half portion of food. I was able to bring the boxed half home to eat the next day. It worked very well for me, and I continue to use that technique time and time again.

Two

Whenever I used to drive to the store (even Target), I would spend up to 15 minutes looking for a parking space as close to the front door as possible. As you can guess, I didn't want to walk any further than necessary to get in the store and get what I needed. All that driving around wasted time, wasted gas and wasted my most precious asset: my **motivation**. Soon, I learned once I started my **One-Step-at-a-Time** process that parking on the far side of the store's lot provided with several benefits. It gave me a chance to spend a few minutes to walk and clear my head before I went in to shop. I found I actually had time to think clearly about what I wanted or didn't want from the store. I was always sure to find plenty of parking, and I never faced a line of cars vying for the same single parking space. My stress levels reduced. It gave me a feeling that I had plenty of time. But most importantly, it gave me a small sense of accomplishment. I walked!

Three

Before you head out for dinner, have a snack. Eat some fruit or a little cheese. A protein bar can also be a good option. A few slices of deli meat can go a long way. Another option is a spoonful of peanut butter. The snack helps curb the appetite and makes you feel more comfortable at the dinner table. The last thing you want to do is step to the table famished. Being overly hungry causes you to fill up on bread, appetizers and a larger dinner than your body needs. Remember it's not just the body that is going to change. It's also the way we think that needs to be adjusted. Trust me, none of us is going to starve by sizing down dinner to a reasonable level. The key to this **One-Step-at-a-Time** process is that **YOU** are making the choices for **YOU**!! You are going to gain control over the different aspects of the battle. **You** get to adjust the rules and customize the tools, tips and practices that are going to help strengthen **YOU**!!

Four

If looking at your scale day after day brings you discomfort, put your scale away for a while. If you have a full-length mirror that you dread walking pass every day, put the mirror away for a while. If you have someone in your life who always wants to talk to you about your weight (other than your doctor or health care professional) and that stresses you out, stop talking to them about your weight and related issues for a while. If you have nothing, but negative self-defeating things to say about yourself, then give the self-talk a rest for a while. The reason I suggest this is to build your confidence. There is no need to continue attacking yourself, bringing yourself down or allowing others to bring you down while you're building up your confidence and strength to fight the war. Give yourself a little time to focus on your steps, use your tips and focus on replacing your bad habits with good ones. The last thing that any of us need is constant reminders of the past we're leaving behind.

Five
There will be times when you get cravings and urges. Make no mistake this war is one that will challenge you. It still challenges me at times. However, I use my tools to fight the good fight. When the urge comes, and it will, the best tool you can employ is time. Time will give you the upper hand over the urge to eat or drink something that you know is not good for you. Do not deny the feeling or urge to eat or drink something, accept it. Accept the urge. Accept the feeling. Don't feel guilty. Don't feel frustrated. Relax. Look at the clock. Give yourself ten minutes. Tell yourself that you will eat or drink it, but not for ten minutes. Those ten minutes will give you a chance to shift the urge into a **decision**. Urges make us do things without really thinking about them. Decisions are made based on our thoughts. Take ten minutes to arm yourself with thought. If ten minutes pass, and you have given it some thought, and you decide that you still want to consume the item then do so. However, have a small portion only then wait another ten minutes. By doing this, you are removing the impulse. Impulse eating or drink is nothing more than acting without thinking. **WE ARE MORE THAN OUR IMPULSES!!!!!** We are thinking, feeling, processing, intelligent human beings and we are taking control of our lives. Build discipline. Build confidence. Begin to trust yourself that you can do this because you are already doing it.

Six

We are human. It's important to remember that when going through the **One-Step-at-a-Time** process. There will be times when life gets the best of us. There will be times when we don't want to get up and get out there. It happens to the best of us. In the past, we've dealt with these feelings in the most negative, and self-destructive ways. We told ourselves we were losers; we couldn't make it; and we shouldn't have started it in the first place. We did our best to tear ourselves down and make sure we never tried again. How dare we even think we could better ourselves? We believed we deserved this life we created. That was the past!!! That was. Now we are going to address what IS!!! We **DO** deserve better! We are better than that! We are making progress! Giving up isn't even an option anymore. The greatest weapon of all: acceptance! When you don't want to get up and start your exercise, accept the feeling. Don't fight the feeling. Don't pretend. Accept it! Relax your mind. Don't pick on yourself about it. Agree with yourself and suit up anyway. Get your walking shoes on anyway. Put on whatever outfit you normally wear anyway. Go outside, or wherever you normally go to exercise and wait five minutes. YES! Suit up, go outside – or to the place you normally do your exercise – and wait five minutes. If five minutes pass and you still don't feel like doing, go back inside and change out of your exercise outfit. One of two things is going to happen. You will either start to exercise or you won't. The battle is in suiting up and getting in to position. That's the real challenge. By doing so, you are sticking to your commitment. If you choose to go back inside and not exercise, at least, you suited up and told yourself you were going through with part of your commitment. That is still a success. If you take the time to suit up and get in to position, most likely, you'll find the courage and motivation to, at least, start the exercise. Once you have started the exercise, chances are you will complete it. Arm yourself! Put on the badge of courage and discipline. You deserve it. You've earned the right to fight the good fight.

"What winning is to me is not giving up, no matter what's thrown at me, I can take it and I can keep going."

Patrick Swayze

Chapter Eight: "From 426 Pounds To The Stage"
Rick Wyckoff

I've struggled with my weight nearly my whole life. In the second grade at just 8 years old, I "ballooned" as my mom used to put it. I was putting on weight so quickly that my parents were buying me new clothes every month. I think I was too young to really grasp what was happening. I mean, I ran track, played soccer, had a swimming pool, biked, climbed trees... did all that and still the weight came on. And so began my epic struggle with my weight.

It's tough growing up and being an overweight kid. I still have very vivid memories of those ridiculing moments when you just feel so isolated and helpless. I mean what's a kid to do? All through junior high and high school I was a pretty lonely teen. I had a few friends who were all overweight. I never took a PE class and avoided that part of campus all together. I remember being intimidated by the athletes and coaches. I would have loved the opportunity to work out, but I just couldn't get myself over there. I mean even as a kid, I wanted to be fit. I wanted to learn more about health and fitness. I wanted to beat the obesity. But I couldn't find any support (of course I never asked) and I never wanted to look like I was unhappy with myself. That was just something else for bullies to attack.

College wasn't quite as bad. People are more into their studies I suppose. Plus being in architecture studio for 100+ hours a week with others, you get to really know people. And I think for the first time, people got to know the real me. I still struggled with my weight and continued to put on weight all through college though.

Even afterwards, having a career, I still hadn't found enough motivation to want to take the weight off.

In August 2004 though, I moved to Alaska. I didn't know anyone up there. I just found a job, an apartment, sold what I couldn't fit into my Toyota Matrix and headed up that way. I figure this would be a great place to kind of make a new start. I was still heavy though. Up there I found out about hiking and biking, 2 of my favorites while I was up there. Also, my brother got married at this time. The pictures from that wedding were enough to get me to do something about my weight. I mean my tuxedo size was "portly." Who the heck came up with that size??? Just another means to mock overweight people? And this started my first REAL attempt at weight loss.

I'm not sure what weight I started out at, but in 2 years I managed to get down to 287 pounds (a loss of around 100 pounds I believe). At first I did at home videos, and "graduated" to the gym, which I have to say was a HUGE accomplishment for me. I was still too shy to lift weights. That's where all the jocks and "bullies" were. So I stayed on the treadmill and elliptical. After the 2 years though, I lost my mojo. I got depressed and numb. I was in denial I was gaining weight back, but my clothes were getting tight (darn washer and dryer!) and I never would step on the scales.

In September of 2010, I moved back down to the lower 48. At this time I was probably at my highest weight ever. Which I'm not real sure, but I'm guessing around 450 pounds. The trip down was incredible, but I couldn't enjoy as much as I would have wanted to. I remember trying to walk up to the rim of Crater Lake and being completely winded. I would have loved to hike while in Yosemite, but I just couldn't. Fitting into a friend's car in Sacramento was so embarrassing for me! And through all that I STILL wasn't motivated to lose the weight. I even walked a 5k in San Antonio at well over 400 pounds.

I started developing anxiety. Simple things like restaurant seats and booths scared me (I've actually broke a couple chairs before). Seat belts in cars scared me, what if I couldn't fit in the seat belt? Chairs during client meetings, clothes at big and tall stores, walking to meetings or with clients somewhere, climbing ladders for my job, just falling over dead from a heart attack. All these were becoming huge sources of fear and anxiety. I finally ended up having an anxiety attack during a staff meeting one day. I couldn't sit still any longer and had no idea what was wrong with me. I couldn't control my heart rate or this weird feeling welling up in me. I excused myself and went to the ER. It took nearly half an hour of me pacing up and down the hall before anyone would see me. When they did my blood pressure was 190/120. They took me in the back and gave me some medication. Eventually my blood pressure went down some, but I had to go see my doctor to get a prescription for anxiety. Even that event though, wasn't enough to get me to change things.

It wasn't until February 13, 2012 that I had my moment. And of all things, it was a pizza binge. I had a bad day at work and came home to my normal therapy at the time, pizza. I downed an entire large pizza, cinnamon sticks, and 2L of soda. For some reason, the rush of being that full just seemed to melt the problems away. But needless to say, I was up sick that night with indigestion. I lay in my bed and just started thinking, what am I doing? My life is becoming a waste. I deserve more than this. Those thoughts just kept repeating themselves in my head.

I woke up the next morning with a new found determination. I got online and researched what I could regarding health and fitness. Things I could do to start the weight loss at 426 pounds. I even looked for pills and shakes and stuff. I also watched some motivational videos of guys who lost a significant amount of weight and one in particular stood out. Eli Sapharti was nearly 300 pounds and in this video, he looked like a fitness model. It just struck me the incredible change. He mentioned that it was his goal to help others achieve their weight loss goals. So I contacted him through an email. And he decided to take me on as a client of his. I remember the first conversation I had with him on the phone. I got something caught in my throat just as he said Hello? And I couldn't say a word and started coughing. He hung up and I thought, oh no there went my opportunity! Luckily he called back and we got off on the right foot hah... literally! He had me walking by the end of that first day. We decided the best approach would be to walk for 15 minutes every day for a week and give up fast food, which I was a fast food nut... at least 3 times a day! So I took on his challenge. I even through in an extra minute just to show him how serious I was about this. The next week, we added 5 minutes and I gave up soda. We used this as a foundation to build a new healthy lifestyle for me, one that was completely sculpted just for me, to work with my life.

Starting out was tough. I expected the cravings and the "not wanting to work out" but I was able to push through that. What I didn't expect was the mocking and the lack of support I would receive. I think the idea of weight loss has become so cliché and almost a waste of an investment that people just scoff at others who "fall victim" to those weight loss scams. I would take my healthy food to work. I would eat my own lunch instead of what a vendor may have brought. People would ask me how I could live on rabbit food and let me know how wonderful the doughnuts and brisket was that I wasn't eating. Sure it was all "in fun" but man, it made it difficult. However, with progress comes change. Not only change in myself, but change in others. As people began to see that I was losing weight, their mockery turned into encouragement, and their scoffs into questions. At my 100 pound weight loss milestone, my office even threw me a party, healthy snacks and all, to celebrate.

My journey's had its ups and downs. It's had its moments where I could have given up. I ended a relationship, I moved from one state to another, celebrated holidays and family reunions. All those could have derailed me, but I kept plowing through. One thing my coach did for me early on was challenged me to run a 5k. I accepted. We slowly started to introduce jogging into my routine... very slowly. At first I could jog no more than 10 seconds at a time. But ya know, I kept at it. Weeks went by and I could jog a whole minute. Months went by and I could jog a mile. Finally I jogged my first 5k in just over an hour. I was so stoked! But knew that I needed to improve my time. There's always something to improve! So from that time, to the race, I worked on my pace and ended up running the 5k race (through sand) at just over 35 minutes. I also got to meet my coach for the first time, and he ran right beside me the entire time, encouraging me every step. It was one of the most awesome experiences of my life.

Eli also encouraged me to start a webpage... www.facebook.com/ConstructingANewRick. It's been humbling, empowering, and life changing. I originally started it as a means of staying accountable to a few people, but it has become so much more than that. The amount of support I receive on there is incredible. Not only from overweight people who see me as an inspiration, but fitness athletes and bodybuilders who say that I inspire them? Me of all people!!! The athletes that I've avoided since I was a kid are on my side and are some of my staunchest supporters. It's been completely eye opening for me to know the positivity that is in the fitness community, and it's something I want to be a part of now.

I have had my share of problems that have arrived during my journey. First and foremost being just sticking with it. There are times when the motivation isn't there. The "newness" of the journey wears off. The only thing that keeps you going sometimes is just being disciplined. Doing what you know you need to do, even though you don't want to. The bad times are fleeting though. Just stick with the routine and before long, you'll be feeling good again. It's amazing how doing things that you know you need to be doing can be empowering and encouraging. You feel better about yourself. Another obstacle is food cravings. I still to this day have cravings that seem beyond control. But there are a few things I've learned you can do to tame them. Eat every 2.5 to 3 hours during the day. This keeps you from being so hungry that you start to make bad decisions. Have an alternative healthy snack available for when you get those cravings. Drink lots of water, especially for those late night cravings. Amazingly, for me, drinking more water throughout the day really does calm those late night cravings. Lastly, K.I.S.S.! Keep It Simple Silly!!! There is a TON of information regarding nutrition and exercise out there. It's important to realize that all you need to really do to get started is just make a slow transition to eating healthier foods and ease into exercise. Just like I did. I started by giving up fast food and walking 15 minutes. Nothing complicated bout that.

Today at 12 months into my journey, I have lost 180 pounds. I've gone from size XXXXXL shirts to XL and size 60 jeans to size 38. In the last few months, I've hired a trainer to help me understand nutrition and exercise more. He has continued to push my intensity in the gym and has helped me take my fitness up a level. Right now I'm working out 2x a day, 5x a week, with cardio in the mornings and resistance training in the evenings. I still have a long road ahead to achieve my goals, but my journey has only just begun. I'm absolutely loving this lifestyle and the results and I'm not about to let anything stop me from it! **NOW IT'S YOUR TURN!!!!**

"Success is to
be measured
not so much by
the position
that one has
reached in life
as by the
obstacles which
he has
overcome."

Booker T. Washington

Chapter Nine: The Bottom Line

Jason: Rick's story was very compelling. I can see how your positive coaching was a perfect fit for his desire to stop the yo-yo-ing and get serious about his health. It's interesting to hear another person's perspective about growing up overweight. When I was a young man, I was very much into sports. I was on the soccer team, ran track and played football. There were kids of all sizes on the teams; I don't think I ever stopped to imagine what the bigger kids were going through. I'm sure I was guilty too of not taking the time to speak with compassion to those overweight kids. I would dare to say I was too caught up in my own insecurities to think about someone else's. I am thankful for you and for Rick to bring these issues out and for being so comfortable talking about those uncomfortable moments in the past. I would assume not everyone has had the results you and Rick have though.

Eli: You are right. In fact, many people have approached me questioning my methods. I have had naysayers my entire life, both before and after I started my journey to better health.

Jason: What are some of the criticisms?

Eli: Jason, I've heard it all. Some have been polite and simply told me my teachings were not for them. Others have been a bit more aggressive, questioning my motives. Some have taken it a step further and attempted to attack my character and tell me I am not qualified to coach. They've told me I don't have a degree in nutrition or a master's degree in sports psychology. If you can imagine it, someone has most likely said it to me at one time or another.

Jason: How do you deal with the criticism?

Eli: I deal with it with compassion.

Jason: Compassion?

Eli: Yes. I deal with them with the same compassion I would want someone to show me. Jason, you have to understand, and I think you are already starting to. Weight is a very personal issue for most people. Being overweight can be directly tied to a person's self-esteem. There are so many people out there that are hurting. These people feel terrible inside because of how they look like on the outside. Add to that a host of *fly-by-night-get-skinny-quick* schemes, that can be both expensive and sometimes dangerous and you get a large group of people upset, skeptical, fed up, angry, resentful and sick and tired of failure.

What they don't understand is, I used to be one of them. I understand. I understand completely. I know what all of those feelings are like. I know what the diet pills, amped up with caffeine, taste like. I know what the walk/jog/running machine in the living room that ends up as a closet to hang clothes looks like. I know what the first day in the gym 100+ pounds overweight feels like. I know how it is to be literally afraid to look down at the scale. It sucks. It's a horribly desperate feeling. This the reason I respond to criticism with compassion. This is why I created a program, a way of attacking the issue of my own weight with my simple **One-Step-at-a-Time** approach.

There is a reason I recommend starting off with very small changes in diet and exercise. There is a reason I recommend suiting up even when one doesn't feel like walking. There's a reason for the motivational quotes. The reason is that it worked for me. Those people attacking me are correct in part. I am not a doctor. I recommend/insist that everyone visit their doctor BEFORE they start working out or making changes to their diet. I am not a health care professional or a health guru. It's very simple. I'm a guy who was way overweight and needed to make a change. I taught myself how to use what I had around me to get started. I was able to achieve some incredible results, results that I believe almost anyone can achieve if they take the time to build up their discipline and confidence.

I'm not angry at those who have expressed antagonism. I have compassion for anyone in the struggle with weight. I make no claims to know it all or to have solved the age-old question of how to get the weight off and keep the weight off for good. That question is up to you to answer. I am here simply to tell the way I was able to achieve MY results. I am here to tell the way some other folks who tried my **One-Step-at-a-Time** process to get the weight off and keep it off.

At the end of the day, it is going to come down to **YOU!** **DO YOU WANT TO GET THE WEIGHT OFF?** Do you want to learn methods that have been proven successful for me and the people I have worked with? Do **You** want to do the work to get the results? I cannot want it for **You**. **You** have to want it for yourself. **You** have to do the walking. **You** have to make the changes in your diet. I am here as a resource. I am here to tell you how I was able to do it. I urge you to ask yourself: **Do You Want It?**

Jason: I have a confession to make. Since we've been working on this book together I have been paying much closer attention to what foods I have been eating, the portions I eat and how often I put in a little exercise.

Eli: That's great! You see, it isn't the hardest thing in the world to do if you just start small.

Jason: That's exactly what I've been telling myself. I've just been taking baby steps. Now, whenever I can, I take the stairs instead of waiting for the elevator. I've really cut down on desserts. But the biggest change of all has been the easiest change to make. I started cooking!

Eli: You weren't cooking before this?

Jason: Nope! Almost every meal, I ate out. I hated cooking. But now I discovered that, by cooking, I can control everything that goes into my meal. I don't have to drive all over town, or wait for a delivery person to show up with my food, and as an added bonus, I've saved an incredible amount of money!!! I don't know why I didn't start cooking a long time ago.

Eli: You see it isn't about changing the world overnight. It's all about making small changes, one at a time, and allowing your mind to register the changes as **good things.** Once your mind understands that **YOU CARE** about your health; it's going to start helping you find ways to improve your health. Once you start finding ways to improve your health, you'll start to see the physical results. Once you start seeing the physical results of your efforts, you'll make great gains in your motivation. Each step supports the next. The most important step is the first. Making that mental decision to **COMMIT** to change is the key to it all. You already made that commitment. You even put it in writing. That decision is one to be proud of and build on. If you have read this far in the book then, obviously, you are still very interested in having a healthier lifestyle. You can do it!! You already started the process.

As the book continues, we will start to address PROGRESS. If, at any time, the book gets ahead of you (meaning that you're still walking 5-15 minutes a day), that's no problem. You're going to catch up at your own pace. You are **NOT** going to move at my pace. Your success is built around creating your **OWN** rules, not following mine. This book is to serve as a resource, not as another ruler to measure either success or failure. I do not believe in that. I believe in taking things as slowly as need be. I believe in doing things in steps and stages. I believe in my **One-Step-at-a-Time** process. I am encouraging you to design a program of exercise and diet that allows you to be human. None of us are perfect, and at the same time all of us are perfect. We have in us all that we need to succeed.

My only expectation is that you learn to be **KIND** to yourself. Being kind to yourself does not mean eating four large pizzas for dinner. It means working with yourself and your personality to create a system of beliefs that allow you to understand that it is okay to succeed. It is through how you treat yourself that you will learn your real value. I can tell you without any doubt in my mind that you are valuable, you are important, you **DO** matter, and you can change **IF** you want to. The tools are here. The motivation is already in you. The desire is inside you just waiting to get out. Allow that desire to get out. Allow yourself be the person that you have always wanted to be, but have been afraid to be. That person is in you right now! Right at this very moment, there is a healthy, fit person inside you waiting to come out and shine.

Let these be the words that reach you to show you that this is your time. This is the moment that you have been telling yourself would come. I would never ask you to do anything I haven't done myself. I found my time in the mirror in Honduras, and I took it. Of course, I had my ups and downs, but the decision and the commitment stayed with me. Join me in the process to get and stay as healthy as possible. Your success grounds me in my own journey and lifts me out of my own struggles. We are far stronger together than we can ever be apart. We are all in this together. That's the bottom line.

"If everyone is moving forward together, then success takes care of itself."

Henry Ford

Chapter Ten: So Now What?

We have come a long way at this point. You set goals and began your own journey. You heard personal stories of overcoming challenges. *So now what?*

Now what **IS** the key. *Now what* is often the difference between whether things happen or not. *Now what* is often the difference between keeping the weight off and settling down on the couch, eating the half-gallon of ice cream on your lap, and fading into the glorious land of *I tried.*

So here is the *Now What!* It's time now to (if you haven't already) immerse yourself into your new **One-Step-at-a-Time** lifestyle. The world feeds you whatever you ask for. You ask for things with your mouth, eyes, ears, heart, and thoughts. Now is the time to get your senses aligned with your overall goal. The goal here is getting healthy. For some of you, this may be for the first time in your entire lives. This may be your first real journey toward getting in shape. For others, this may be time #7,346. It doesn't matter. Once you see the weight start to drop and your energy increase, it is time to add to your momentum.

Most of us have a few spare minutes in our busy day. Some of us have more than a few minutes throughout the day to allow our thoughts, and sometimes our bodies to wander. It's time to reel that time in. Going forward, it's very important to fill those empty minutes with conscious thought and action. What do I mean by that? I mean start to study!! If you were in school, you would have classroom time and homework. You would have to study to instill your consciousness with the subject. The teacher would assign you reading material, practical application projects, and test you to make sure you absorb the material. This isn't much different, except YOU are going to create the lesson, textbooks, and tests for yourself.

When free time presents itself, USE IT!!! READ!! Start using the internet to research stories of success. Learn about healthy food and ways to prepare it that works with your body. Retrain your brain to see that jock, or that girl with the *perfect body*, are not aliens from Mars. They are where you are headed. Of course, you don't have to end up as an Olympic athlete, or a swimsuit model to have succeeded. But you will accomplish your goals of losing weight and getting healthy.

Take inventory of the magazines you have in your house. Write down what TV shows you like to watch. What websites you browse? What are you surrounding yourself with at this current moment? Do you have healthy images on the screensaver of your computer? What pictures do you have on the door of your fridge? THESE THINGS MATTER!!! It matters what you see, hear, touch and feel. These things shape the way you think!! We are products of our environment. Let's clean house and set up an environment to help us!!!!

If you're going to take the time to read, why not read stories about successful journeys to weight loss and good health? If you're going to watch TV, and you insist on watching a food channel; watch a channel that focuses on healthy cooking. Cut out a few pictures of the new healthy and delicious foods you're going to try. Hang those pictures on the fridge. If you find yourself near a mall, pull in. Remember to park far enough away for a nice relaxing walk to the entrance. Rather than hanging your head while walking into the *Big and Tall* shop, lift your chin and walk into the shoe store and size up your next pair of walking shoes. Those shoes may soon become jogging shoes, those jogging shoes, running shoes!!!!!

This next topic is very important. I might go so far as to say it may be the difference between *getting it,* and *NOT getting it.* SO if you don't have time to concentrate right now, put down the book. Come back to it later.

The time has come for **You** to support **You**. The time to feel shame about yourself is finished. The time to feel joy and self-esteem about your body has arrived. The idea of the rude insensitive comments we've all heard having any value has now passed. This is a new age. This is the time to tune out the hecklers, forgive the ignorant, surpass the limitations, and rise above. This is the time you are going to allow you to feel good about yourself and what you are doing now. The past is called the past for a reason. It's because we have already passed it by. It is behind us for a reason. It's behind us so that we don't have to look at it as we travel forward. This is the moment to agree with that part of yourself that always told you that you are good enough, and that you do deserve a better life. You deserve a healthier life. You deserve more energy. You deserve to smile when you look in the mirror. You are greater than any number on a scale. You are one of a kind, and you are on a journey towards your goals. Just because you are on that journey, success is already yours!! The limitations, placed on you by the world are there to test you. They are in place to trip you up and hold you down. I am here to tell you that you are greater than the roadblocks in front of you and greater than the potholes behind you.

So many people told me I couldn't do it. In fact, I may have been the one speaking the loudest about my assured failure. I had myself convinced. It was what it was, and there was very little I could do about it. **I THOUGHT!!!** Looking back on it now, it's not that hard to see why I stayed the way I was for so damn long. How could I have expected my body to change when my mind was made up? Think about it! I couldn't even escape a Target. How in the world was I going to be able to escape a self-imposed prison of food, fat and complacency? I was that little voice in my head saying, *"Eli, you aren't good enough. Eli, you will never be fit. Eli, you are trapped. Eli, the journey is too far; just have another pizza. Eli, you are too fat to run. You are too fat to even begin. Eli, all those people were right. You are a gordo, you are a bubble butt, and you are a fatso!!! Have another slice. Let me get you some extra dressing. You know that little plate is not going be enough. Hell yeah! You want cake! Get a bigger glass. You want to super-size that?"*

ENOUGH

ENOUGH

ENOUGH

ENOUGH

It really is enough! Those voices need addressing. Those voices need a confrontation. Those voices need changing. You do have the right to be! You do have the right to avoid the foods that are not good for you. You do have the right to exercise. You do have the right to succeed. It is your time to shine. It is your time to walk down the sidewalk, unconcerned about your size. It is time to add some pep to your step. This is that day. This is that time. You can do this. And I will take it a step further and tell you directly that you ARE DOING THIS!!! It has already begun. **You** are your teacher. **You** are your coach. **You** are your trainer. **You** are already making progress!!

Bring these thoughts with you when you're walking, at your job, and driving your car: *I have finally made the decision that is changing my life one step at a time. Although I am not perfect, I am perfectly ME. I am doing the things I need to do, to become the healthier, happier and more confident ME. I cannot change other people, but I can measure them by the kindness they display, or the cruelty of their actions. No matter what they or anyone else says, I know that I am on the right track. I may stumble; everyone does. I may fall as many have fallen before me. However, no matter what I do, I have committed myself to getting back up, dusting myself off, and continuing my journey. I am not in a contest with anyone else. I am not here to impress anyone, other than myself. I am here to take this journey **One Step at a Time**. I am here to be. I am worth the time. I am worth the work and I am worth the results. This is the beginning of a new relationship with **ME!!***

"Love yourself first and everything else falls into line. You really have to love yourself to get anything done in this world."

Lucille Ball

Chapter Eleven: Finding Your Fun

Jason: So where do you want to go from here? We have taken the reader on a journey through the first steps. We have addressed habits, emotional pitfalls, discipline, self-esteem and heard part of your testimony, as well as Rick's.

Eli: Now I want to talk about a word few people associate with health and fitness. **FUN!**

Jason: Fun?

Eli: Yes, **FUN.** Going through the **One-Step-at-a-Time** process can be tiring, tedious, painful and embarrassing. However, once the ball starts rolling, and you make a little progress, it can also be FUN. When I began the process, I was a mess. I had little or no energy and even less motivation. I hated the way I looked and judged myself minute by minute. I was, by far, my worst critic. But once I reached a certain point, the walking became routine. The items in my diet became less painful to replace. I actually began feeling a little pride in my progress.

Jason: That sounds excellent.

Eli: Yes, but I needed to keep things fresh. I'm easily bored. I know myself pretty well, and I knew that once I was able to walk for15 minutes, I needed to bump it up to 20 minutes. 20 minutes became 30 and so on. I knew I needed a new challenge. So I started jogging **One Step at a Time.** First, I jogged for a minute returned to walking then jogged for two minutes. It didn't take long for my 30-minute walk to turn into a 30-minute jog.

111

Jogging eventually turned into running. Running turned into racing: 2K, 5K, 10K and the half-marathon. Now I'm considering a full marathon. I continue to push myself. I challenge myself to keep my mind active and find the FUN in staying healthy. Without the FUN, exercise and proper diet feels more like punishment.

Jason: Are you suggesting that people reading this book make running a marathon as a goal?

Eli: No! Running was my choice. Everyone has different interests, and is looking for different results. For **ME,** running works. For others, it may not.

Jason: Basically the reader needs to find their own passion?

Eli: EXACTLY!!!! That is exactly what I am saying. For some, it may be running. For others, it may be a kick-boxing class. I have a client who loves to cycle. I encourage my clients to find what they really ENJOY doing. We are not all the same, and we don't all like the same activities. Finding your own passion will help you gain control over your life and your health. This is a journey, and it's meant to be fun as well as liberating. Here are some activities a person can look into: walking, speed-walking, stair-climbing, jogging, swimming, spinning, cross-fit, kayaking, weightlifting, biking, and paddle-boarding to name a few. If they find a match, perfect! If they don't, then they can keep looking.

Jason: So immersing oneself in information was leading up to this?

Eli: Right again! You see you're starting to get it. By reading, posting pictures of healthy ideas, foods, and routines, you are encourage yourself to Think Healthy. We have to make ourselves comfortable with the idea of a healthy lifestyle BEFORE we can have one. Once we see what it looks like, it makes it much easier to pursue. Taking control of the process, customizing it to one's likes gives the person even more reason to get out there, and put some passion into their workout. Trust me; few things are more painful or emotionally draining than loathing a workout and suiting up to do it *one more time*. It feels like a prison. I don't want to imprison people; I want to set them free. That is my whole goal. I am successful because I started with a realistic approach to solving problems. I have a deep understanding of how hard it is to get motivated, and to STAY motivated. Losing weight and gaining energy, and getting fit and staying fit looks great on paper. But to do it, to get out there and make a real and lasting change can be, for some, the hardest thing they have ever faced in life.

Jason: How does it feel to help people and to teach people how to help themselves?

Eli: How does it feel to write your books?

Jason: It's the greatest gift I have been given to date.

Eli: I couldn't have said it better myself!!

Jason: In the last chapter, we spoke about readers immersing themselves into the mental and visual idea of a healthy life. Now we are getting into customizing the daily workout routine. I assume the readers' diet is also customizable?

Eli: Definitely! Billions of dollars are spent marketing *diet food* to potential consumers each year. Every day, we are flooded with commercials, magazines, and radio ads. There are a million messages for the next best thing to make the pounds fall away. Pills, potions, diet snacks, and pre-packaged meals are all around us. Those things can be great if the consumer believes in them. I try not to discourage anyone from doing something that works to promote a healthier lifestyle. I believe in personal freedom rather than telling someone what to eat and where to shop to get in shape. I, however, did not find the success I was looking for in these products. I found that a healthy diet, implemented over time, was the most successful route for me to take.

Jason: I assume you tried quite a few before coming to that conclusion?

Eli: I felt like I tried them all, Jason. I would've eaten a shoe if I thought it would help me get anywhere with my weight. But I wasn't learning anything by consuming those products.

Jason: What do you mean?

Eli: I mean, I wasn't learning **HOW** to eat. I was only being told **what** to eat. Through research into learning what foods work with my body and what foods don't, I was able to UNDERSTAND what I need and what I don't. You see, I involve myself, and give myself a much greater sense of control over my future and my destiny. I prepare my food. I know exactly what is going into my body. I avoid processed food. I choose the natural ingredients my body needs. When I ordered a pizza, or unwrapped a microwave dinner, I put almost no thought into what was going in my body. Food was a phone call, or a few buttons on the microwave screen. Boom! Dinner! Done! I didn't give it a second thought. Now it's a totally different experience. I see what's going into the pan. I choose every single item. I customize the menu, and I love it. Not only do I end up with a healthy, tasty, colorful meal, but I actually enjoy the process of choosing. The time spent paying close attention to what goes into my body increases my pride, health, and joy of my spirit. It also increases my total commitment to my goal.

Jason: Choosing?

Eli: Choosing! It is one of the greatest ways I show myself that I care about myself.

"You can search throughout the entire universe for someone who is more deserving of your love and affection than you are yourself, and that person is not to be found anywhere. You yourself, as much as anybody in the entire universe deserve your love and affection."

Buddha

Chapter Twelve: Jennifer

I've struggled with weight since puberty, which came pretty early for me. I was an active kid, a bit of a Tomboy in fact, one that you would find outside on the school playground running, jumping, climbing anything I could. Then at age nine, I had a huge growth spurt, hit puberty, and so began my battle with weight. Talk about a shock to the system, it's tough for a kid to go from fitting in to being one of the tallest kids in the 4th grade, let alone being a girl starting to develop into a woman, yet still wanting to run around on the playground like a child.

Going from elementary school into junior high, the struggle only became worse as I continued to put on more weight. In seventh grade, I tried out and actually made the school's drill team. I was probably the chubbiest one of the bunch. I recall begging my mom to sew my uniform because buying one from the store was next to impossible as they didn't exactly come in my size. Needless to say, changing in the girls locker room made me loathe my PE class, so I would find very creative ways to avoid it all together to the extent that I'd get in trouble for not changing into my gym clothes. I always had a great group of friends, yet as we all started to grow up and mature into teens, my self-esteem continued to plummet. And let me tell you, hearing from your loved ones about how pretty your face is and how if you would only lose weight, does not make you feel better one bit, at least it did nothing but make me feel like a failure. I purposely missed out on numerous teenage rites of passage like going to prom so as not to feel even worse about myself, other kids can be so cruel. I could not wait to get out of high school! My self-esteem had gotten so bad that I went from being a student who excelled at just about every subject, especially math, was in all the advanced placement classes and had a pretty great GPA, to one that started to cut class and eventually school altogether. In my senior year, I begged our assistant principal to allow me to attend a continuation school for a semester so I could get caught up and essentially make up all the missing credits I now needed to graduate. Luckily, I was granted this request, complied with my part of the agreement and returned to the regular school in time to graduate with my class. I'll never forget how disappointed my family was that I was not up there graduating with honors, while I was happy that I at least graduated "on-stage" with my class, my self-worth was completely shot.

I had started working at a very young age, so it was relatively easy for me to land great full-time jobs as a young adult. I went to college, worked full-time and began to lead a pretty active social life. It was fantastic, being in the real world with adults, I finally felt like I could be my true self and that people liked me, despite my weight problem. I began going out quite often, which involved all kinds of temptation. That's also when my yo-yo dieting began. I attempted every diet imaginable, Weight Watchers, Jenny Craig, various shady "diet clinics" offering versions of Phen-fen, Atkins, Lindora. You name it I "tried" ALL of them. Guess what, they all worked – temporarily. I would lose, gain, lose and ultimately regain the same 30 – 40 pounds over and over and over again, each time adding just a little bit more.

As an adult, my weight fluctuated between, the heaviest I can remember, 269lbs to the lowest right around

200lbs. Every New Year, I would make that same resolution... THIS would be the year! I was going to lose all the weight. Well, in January of 2008, as most enjoyed a long weekend in observance of the MLK Jr. Holiday. I decided I would empty out my storage unit and enlisted the help of a friend. I remember it so vividly, as we were moving some items and loading them onto his truck, I nearly passed out! My friend was concerned, I could tell, but he tried to play it off by making a joke that I was trying to get out of doing any heavy lifting.

As he followed me in his truck, I called to tell him I needed pull over to get something to drink right away, my mouth was so incredibly dry and I felt completely parched, it was the weirdest feeling ever. We chalked it up to the salty Chinese food we had eaten the previous night. That same weekend, I had another near fainting experience. After spending the long weekend feeling terrible, weak, light headed, extremely thirsty, I knew something just wasn't right. First thing that Tuesday, I made a phone call and was able to squeeze in to see an associate of my regular physician. Within 10 minutes of walking into his office that afternoon, I had been diagnosed as Type 2, Diabetic with a blood glucose of nearly 400 and an A1c of 10. There I was, 37 years old, my weight had ballooned to 270lbs, and no known history of diabetes in my family. I did this to myself!!! I remember leaving the medical clinic in tears, terrified, thinking I was going to live a miserable existence and probably die young.

This was it, my moment. What was I going to do now??? Well being scared to death can really motivate one to change; at least it did for me. I realized there was no more time to waste and I needed to take action. For the next 5 months I cut out virtually ALL bad carbs, sugars, sweets, sodas, etc. - even alcohol, which was extremely difficult for my social life. I truly focused on myself for once and pretty intensely I might add, to the degree that I withdrew from my life. By the time my June birthday rolled around, 2008; I had lost 60 lbs. All naturally, no magic pills or shortcuts – except for my diabetes medication of course that I had to now take. I did tons of research, read books, magazines and lots of online research tested my blood glucose daily – OUCH! Those lancets can really hurt after so many pricks. I actually used my gym membership, what a novel idea, right? I learned what to eat and what spiked my blood glucose levels. My doctor was impressed with my A1c which is a blood test, also known as Hemoglobin A1c, it provides an average of your blood sugar control over a six to twelve week period. My results had gone from an A1c of 10 to nearly 5. The doc agreed, I seemed to have things under control and took me off my medications. What a relief! Was I cured? Was it possible to CURE this disease that has overtaken our society?

In the comfort of knowing I would 'live" I began to ease up on my short-lived, extreme, new existence. It was only natural, for almost 6 months prior I felt I was hardly "living" at all on that plan. There I was again, the point I had reached several times before. I was back in my comfort zone, hovering just above/below the 200lb mark. I looked pretty good! My "skinny clothes" fit again. For whatever reason, perhaps genetics, I tend to carry my weight evenly and surprisingly don't appear to weigh as much as I actually do, could also be the fact that I always wear heels too, lending to that illusion. Much to my dismay and before I realized it, the lifestyle that had originally gotten me to my lowest point early in

120

2008 had slowly crept back in. I guess there truly may not be a real cure for what I had. I started to feel bad again physically and had regained nearly 40lbs. Back I went on those diabetes meds.

My teens, twenties, and now thirties had all gone by and at 40 years old, I was FINALLY ready to take FULL control of my life, health & happiness. I had let myself "go" for the last time, weighing in at 239.9, after all, every ounce counted I hadn't yet gotten back to 240! On January 14th of 2012, four years into my Type 2 diagnosis, I said ENOUGH IS ENOUGH! It was time. I knew what to do. I knew it worked. I NEEDED to stay focused! I needed to change my life and stop going on a "diet". A true lifestyle change is what I needed, nothing temporary.

A lifelong friend of mine was on a similar path. She had started following a bunch of what I called "fitness freaks" on Facebook. I was pretty resistant to doing anything of the sort. I didn't need anyone's help. I know what to do, and I can do this on my own! Yes I can be pretty darn stubborn. Well thankfully she would let me rant, and then she'd answer my questions about the whole thing afterward. My friend mentioned a few motivational types she was following and in that she told me there was even a guy, somewhere in Florida, that had lost a LOT of weight and he would post all this wonderful inspirational/motivational stuff. I had to check it out for myself.

Eli Sapharti – Fat Boy Fit Man, I found him! Wait, that can't be true, here's a guy who weighed 300 lbs. and now looked like a fitness model? What is THIS all about? What did he DO? How can I do that and get to MY own goals? These were all questions in my head of course. I began to follow Eli's Facebook page. His posts were truly inspirational. He was talking about things that made sense, not just trainer type advice as in, do this or that to get results, but more about changes that come from within. I couldn't wait any longer I needed to know what to do to finally get THERE! I contacted Eli and he took me on as a client. His advice, encouragement and support inspired me to keep moving on in my own journey, he's taught me to stop settling and keep marching forward towards my goals. I have lost over 100 lbs. and am currently at my lowest adult weight ever. My diabetes is now under control WITHOUT any medication whatsoever. Those A1c results? For nearly one year, they have consistently ranged from 4.5 – 5.0. This is considered "normal" vs. diabetic. My doctor has said to me that if I continue this way for the next 6-12 months he will remove the Type 2 Diabetes from my list of "problems". I no longer "black-out" like I used to. I am the happiest, healthiest and SKINNIEST I have been in OVER 20 years, there's NO STOPPING me now!

With Eli's encouragement, I have also started my own fan page: www.facebook.com/SugarFreeandShrinking. I began it with the intention of holding myself accountable and avoid any backsliding, now that I have all these followers, I have to keep going! What an incredible experience, there are so many amazingly supportive folks out there also looking for that missing piece it seems. There are many of us Looking for a little extra daily push or sharing tips that we have all learned and continue to learn along the way. This journey for me is so much more than the numbers on a scale. It's more than getting healthy and getting off medication and being able to stop pricking my fingers on purpose every day. It has done wonders for my self-esteem and self-worth and is spilling over into all the areas of my life. This has been a true journey in self-discovery. I know and can accept that I am not perfect, there is no such thing. Just be realistic. I set my goals. I am consistent and if I falter, don't beat myself up. I get right back up and keep going. I put one foot in front of the other and One Step at a Time. The sky is the limit!

- Jennifer Babsky

"Your time is limited, so don't waste it living someone else's life. Don't be trapped by dogma - which is living with the results of other people's thinking. Don't let the noise of others' opinions drown out your own inner voice. And most important, have the courage to follow your heart and intuition."

Steve Jobs

Chapter Thirteen: Internal

Jason: Another compelling story of success!

Eli: Jennifer has been very dedicated to her progress, and seeing the benefits has only strengthened her resolve.

Jason: That's got to be a great feeling for you as well.

Eli: It is. Seeing my clients overcome their internal limitations and begin the journey to healthy living strengthens me. And now would be a good time to talk about some of the health benefits that Jennifer and others have experienced by improving what they eat and losing weight.

Jason: I'm not a doctor, but I can imagine losing weight through exercise and eating right are two of the best things you can do for yourself.

Eli: They are. I am not a doctor either. I mentioned this several times already in the book. I cannot stress it enough. Constant communication with one's doctor or health care professional is key, when beginning and throughout this journey. There can be major risks to unhealthy people starting a new exercise routine. Changing your diet when you're on medications can also be very risky. I, by no means, want to imply that losing weight will bring you total health, and cure all of your ills. With that being said, I've heard and experienced some amazing stories of success. This book is about the results I have had in my life, and the results of various other individuals, who have shared their stories.

Jason: Wow! That sounds like a pretty serious disclaimer.

Eli: I have learned that there are many litigious people out there looking to place the blame for their shortcomings on others. Although it's very sad; unfortunately, it is also necessary to clarify that everyone's results may be different, and that we are not giving medical advice.

Jason: Duly noted.

Eli: As you can see from Jennifer's story, amazing things can happen when we begin to take our health seriously. Jennifer was able to transform from the edge of a critical medical condition just by changing her diet and establishing and maintaining an exercise routine. But the stories don't stop with Jennifer.

Using my **One-Step-at-a-Time** process, I achieved my initial goal of shedding 110 pounds. But it didn't stop there. The process and the weight loss helped me address many problems, other than the size of my waistband. Back in those days, I also smoked cigarettes like a chimney. I used to sweat profusely, even while walking from my car to my desk at work. I had panic attacks, and my environment was limited to home, work and the nearest Target store. I was tired all the time, and rarely had the energy to get through my daily routine. In addition to my lack of energy, my body was truly paying the price. My joints ached as I was carrying around an extra 110 pounds. For me, just breathing was a challenge. My blood pressure and cholesterol levels were through the roof. I had created a perfect storm to kill myself. There was very little doubt about that. The

126

anxiety from knowing that I was so unhealthy was driving me crazy. Literally!

Things change in life. Sometimes we change them ourselves. Sometimes life changes them for us. In my case, it was a combination of things. Those words from the cashier, the full-length mirror in Honduras, and my freeway panic attack all played a role in my decision to change. In the beginning of the process, I felt as if my physical condition worsened. It didn't. In hindsight, I can see that was just my body reacting to change, change from the inside out. As my confidence grew my anxiety faded a bit. As the pounds dropped off, I began to breathe a little easier. As I began to breathe easier, I pushed myself harder. As I pushed myself harder, I gained more confidence. And as I gained more confidence, I began to feel much better about myself, thus addressing some of my anxiety and depression. I created an unexpected chain reaction. To my surprise, my blood pressure and cholesterol levels started dropping along with the size of my waistband. I could feel the changes happening.

The chain reaction continued. Because my **One-Step-at-a-Time** process dealt with discipline, as well as diet and exercise, I trained my brain and body to do more, want more, and be more than I ever had in the past. My mental game improved, at least, as rapidly as my physical. The exercise gave me better circulation throughout my body. The will to do the exercise circulated positive thoughts throughout my mind. Together the combination built on itself. The more I started to do, the more I wanted to do. **One Step at a Time!**

The chain reaction extended to my emotional life, as well. As I got *healthier*, I got happier. I began to feel more comfortable with myself and, therefore, with other people. My relationships started to improve. I relaxed my defensive nature a bit and became more expressive and comfortable with conversation. I applied my success on the track, in my work, with my family and my friends. It was like living in a jail cell all my life until one day discovering that I had been sitting on the key the entire time! When that cell door open, I gained a new lease on life!!

Of course, I still heard those voices in my head telling me that *I couldn't do it, I wasn't worth it, and I didn't deserve it.* I think we all have those voices. However, I had new voices now, telling me the opposite. ***I could do it; I was doing it, and I was going to continue to do it well into the future!!*** Those positive voices grew louder and louder. With each goal reached, the positive self-talk increased. Even the mirror started to be kind to me. I stopped putting a towel over the scale in the bathroom. My fears began to fade, and a new Eli began to emerge.

The healthy diet and exercise probably saved my life. I know it made massive improvements to my life. And at the end of the day, isn't that what we all want? Aren't we all trying to get a little better than we were the day before? None of us are perfect. None of us are ever going to be perfect. But we can, with a little work and some better decisions, improve. We can set goals and accomplish them. We all have the ability to reach for higher heights, and transform ourselves from people that *try* to people that **DO**. To me, that is what it's all about. It's about doing, being and reaching to be the best you that you can possibly be. Excel! I dare you. I challenge you to reach a little further and see how you feel. Set goals, accomplish them, and pay attention to how you feel. Never be afraid of quitting something that you have started. However, be very afraid of never starting something in the first place. You are the person who determines who you are, how you are, and what you are worth. I cannot do that part for you. That, my dear friend, is totally up to you.

"So what do we do? Anything. Something. So long as we just don't sit there. If we screw it up, start over. Try something else. If we wait until we've satisfied all the uncertainties, it may be too late".

Lee Iacocca

Chapter Fourteen: Getting Back Up

Jason: Very few of us need help falling down. We can manage that all by ourselves. We often set goals and fall short. We often reach for the stars, only to come crashing back to earth like a fiery comet. It's part of life. It's built into the process of success. Even while you are reading this book, you are succeeding with a series of your past failures. You can read the words on this page, right? Have you always been able to read? Even when you were two years old? Learning to read takes years of *not being able to do it*; to actually do it, and read a whole book. It takes time to grow, and in most people's process of growth, there comes the time to dust off after a fall or two.

Many years ago, I was living in the Caribbean when a massive, Category 5 hurricane approached the island. I hadn't had a drink of liquor, at that time, in about ten years. I was scared, very scared. I never experienced a hurricane, let alone a CAT 5. One thing led to another, and before long I was face-to-face with three large bottles of rum. Do you know what I did next? Exactly! I got drunk! In fact, on that day, I started drinking again. I fell off the wagon and on to my chin.

At times, we fall. At times, we fail. Those are the givens. My question to you isn't if, or when you are going to fail at anything in life. My question is very simple: What are you going do about it if, or when you stumble, come up on hard times, or fall short? Are you going to pack up your toys and run home? Are you going to spend the next five years angry with yourself? Are you a blame shopper? I mean, do you search around for the best person, place, or thing to blame your problems on? How do you recover from your setbacks and how can you improve your process of recovery?

Today, I don't drink. Today, Eli is 110 pounds lighter than he was six years ago. If either of us wallowed in the mistakes we had made along the way, we wouldn't be here talking to you today. Disappointments are natural. Rain is natural. No matter how much we love the sun, it's still gonna rain at some point. Do you like flowers? Do you like seeing a beautiful green lawn? How about a beautiful mountain stream, rainbow, or waterfall? All of those things and more come from the rain. When I hear people say, *I hate the rain,*" a smile crosses my face because I know I have just heard a lie.

Eli: What Jason says is true. This has been a journey filled with some high highs and some low lows, but through it all, I have been transforming myself. My experiences are now helping other people. I am able to share my ups and downs with others to help them reach their goals. How would I be able to do this if I was still sitting on my couch, picking on myself because one night I broke my routine, and had a wild romance with an extra-large pizza, a coke and half-gallon of ice cream? I don't think I could. I don't think I would have made it at all until I learned how to get back up.

People! Ask yourself: How many diets so far? I mean, to date. How many diets or programs have you started and stopped? How many times have you worked up the courage to join a gym? How many times have you said, okay, no more junk food? For most of us, the list is long and painful to look at. But I'm here today to tell you that, at least, we started to take steps to improve. The problem lies in quitting then picking on ourselves.

Let me ask you this: If you walked along a grassy trail and, all of a sudden, you slipped and found yourself on the ground, would you get up or just lay there until the end of time? Would you lay there and imagine all the reasons you deserved to lay on the ground, or would you get up and continue walking down the trail? If you got up, would you immediately throw yourself right back down on the ground? Or would you step a bit more carefully while you proceeded down the trail? Imagine for a minute that you continued down the trail, taking in the beauty of nature, when the sharp edge from a broken branch cuts your leg. What are you going to do? Do you take that branch and start cutting your wound over and over? Do you yell at yourself for being so stupid that you fell down, only to get back up to get cut by a branch? These, and more, are the choices you have at your fingertips. How about this: Let's stop the bleeding first. Let's make a mental note that there are sharp branches and objects along the trail, which can trip us up. Then let's use the experience to keep from falling as we go further along the trail.

One night a group of us went out for drinks. I had already lost about 80 pounds, by that the time, and I was feeling pretty good about myself. The drinks started flowing, and before long, I was a little drunk. I think most of us know that when the buzz from alcohol comes on, resistance and discipline tends to go down. Sometimes it goes way down. The next thing I knew, I was at an all-night breakfast joint staring down at a full breakfast platter and a chocolate milk shake. It must have been three or four in the morning. This was a feast with enough calories to fuel my body for days. I buried myself in the meal. I woke up the next day (well, later that morning I should say) and felt terrible. I wanted to beat myself up. I wanted to punish myself. I felt like crap. **BUT!!!** I knew better than to start the self-hating again. I knew better than to stay down. I knew better than to go out and triple my exercise routine in an attempt to cover my tracks. I did none of the above. I sat down for a moment, and just spoke to myself, using words of encouragement and peace rather than beating myself over the head because of a big breakfast and a chocolate shake. I built myself up by telling myself: The night was a mistake and there were things I could have done differently to avoid the end result.

When you're in an environment where you know alcohol is served keep in mind that you may become enticed. If you are going out for just drinks and not dinner, why not prepare a healthy meal before you go? Getting yourself prepared to battle is better than having to defend yourself after the fight has been fought. Once you get to the venue, remember drinks are full of calories. Try to include a glass of water or two between each drink. Know that if you get buzzed or drunk, there is a good chance your resistance to food is going to go down...way down. So think ahead. Look at the menu for some emergency items you can order if you must. Pizza would not be one of those items. I am sorry. Double-loaded twice-baked potatoes would also not make the list. A veggie plate would work but hold the blue cheese and ranch dip. A salad would also work. If you are really hungry, add some grilled chicken to the salad. Though try not to add the double-bacon cheeseburger. Remember this is a battle, and you have tools and weapons to win this fight and the next one and the next one. If a burger or a creamy plate of pasta gets past your shield... deal with it. Address the choice of ordering it, eating it, and the feelings that will come afterward like a fall on the trail. I'm pretty sure the world didn't end the moment you spooned up a gallon of ice cream. It was a choice. It was a lapse in judgment. Get back up as fast as possible and put it behind you.

That doesn't mean do it six nights a week, and put six nights a week behind you. It means keep your self-esteem up and realize that this is a journey. You have signed an agreement with yourself. My name and Jason's name are not on the agreement. **YOUR NAME IS!!!** You agreed to begin this process. This is an ongoing process, and one that can take you from the couch to the finish line.

In some ways, this is the most important chapter of this book. We have all started processes before. We *try*, we lose a little, we fail, and we give up. We *try*, we lose a little, we fail, and we give up. Over and over, we go like a pair of pants spinning around in the dryer. Here is my question: Why? Why do we feel that somehow, we are less deserving than the next person to be healthy, happy and confident in ourselves? Why do we punish ourselves? Why are our dreams somehow less important than everyone else's dreams? Is the weight we carry some crime we have committed? Are we doomed to a life of looking out the window and wishing we were someone else, or had someone else's body? I say: **HELL NO!!!!!** This is a personal prison that we have created, and the key is under our butts! In order to get the key, we have to get off of our butts, pick the key up, walk over to the door of the cell, and put the key into the lock. We need to turn the key, and open the door. That's it. Get up. Get walking. Get out of your cell.

Jason: I couldn't agree more. Whenever I set out on an adventure, or started a new endeavor, I always faced the critics. There are always the voices. They try telling me: *Jason, you can't make it, it won't work, it's too risky, Jason, you aren't prepared, play it safe* and my favorite: *Why do you think you can do it, when so many before you have failed?*

Here's the problem with *the voices*. When they come from outside, I find them much easier to deal with. I can smile and tell the person with doubts about me that I appreciate their concerns. I can be polite to them and just be on my way. **BUT!!!!** When those voices are coming from within, it can be much harder to deal with. I can't be polite to myself and walk out of the room. I am still gonna be with me in the next room!!! So what do I do? How do I address my worst critic...me!! ?? I have to first understand that these inner doubts are nothing more than my own fears of succeeding. These are the same voices that have judged me throughout my entire life and kept me from my greatest victories. Ultimately, I have to recognize that these voices, whether good or bad, work for me. It is not the other way around. I am the boss and they are just voices. I also have to look at my commitment to my progress. I am doing something about my weight, or my bad habits. I am in motion. The voices need to be retrained to my current position. I am no longer a child, a teenager or a twenty-year old. I am no longer my former self. I am growing and I have grown dramatically from what I used to be.

Eli: OK, so you may be facing a lapse in judgment. You may have just come off of an eating binge, and you feel terrible. What do you do? I suggest that you go back to the beginning of the book and re-read the steps. Look at the commitment you have already made with yourself. There you will find the strength and courage needed to dust yourself off, and get right back at it. You do not need to double your efforts, or increase your exercise time, to make up for what's already happened. It's already in the past. Forgive yourself and buckle back into your routine. It has already started working for you. Look at the situation that made you fall and learn from it. Learn how to prevent it from happening a second and third time. You are growing. You are learning about yourself, what works for you, and what doesn't. You have not been hired as your own personal critic. You are a teacher. You are teaching yourself that you can improve; you can reach higher, and you can regroup, and get to it again.

It has taken an incredible amount of practice for me to get where I am. The journey is not over yet. I am still tempted time and time again to slide back, but I've learned how to encourage myself. I have learned what kind of talk I need to have with myself, to push me forward, and not hold me back. I go back to the steps, and look at places I can improve. I ask myself: Can I replace this food with a healthier choice? Can I improve my time in the next race I run? What is my next set of goals? And most importantly... who else can I help?

Jason: This process is about you. This is about you getting real with yourself, and creating a plan that will actually work for you. Our goal is for you to be the best that you can be. We want to empower you by giving you some simple tools to use on your journey. We all set out to do our best. Sometimes we fall. But when we fall, we need to get back up. When we get back up, we need to learn from the past then leave it in the past. Every single day is a brand new day, and no two are alike. Let's make this new day count!!!

"If you accept the expectations of others, especially negative ones, then you never will change the outcome."

Michael Jordan

Chapter Fifteen: Them, They and Those

Eli: There are going to be those people who cannot and will not get past your new desire for a better you. They may say or do any number of things to attempt to throw you off course. That's just them. The them, they, and those of this world will always be there. The thing that may surprise you is how close to home they really are.

On my journey, I experienced all kinds of situations, where people said and did things to me that hurt. Sometimes it was in the form of a joke. Sometimes it was all-out confrontation. In each case, I tried to keep my cool, and allow my own insecurities to pass before I responded.

Jason: Give me an example.

Eli: One of my co-workers ordered doughnuts and urged everyone to have one. I explained that I wasn't eating sweets and the teasing began. *"Oh, come on, Eli, just one isn't going to hurt you. It's just a doughnut. Just one little tiny doughnut is going to ruin your whole diet?"* I recognized that the coworker had no idea how badly I wanted to eat that doughnut, as well as, every other doughnut within a five-mile radius of the building. I had to keep telling myself that she wasn't teasing me to tease me. She just didn't have the food issues I had, and meant no harm.

Jason: Yeah, I have been through the same thing with friends offering me a drink. After I explain for 25 minutes how drinking is different for me than it is for them, they still come back with: *"Dude, I just can't* *believe that you can't even have one drink."* It does get annoying very quickly.

Eli: But, at least, with liquor you can say: *"I am in recovery and I really can't drink."* Imagine saying: *"Guys, I'm in recovery from doughnuts, so please don't offer me any."*

Jason: Excellent point.

Eli: The tool I employed to fight office doughnuts, sugar cookies at the bank, and Sunday afternoon nachos during the football game, was **choice.** I would tell them I'm **choosing** to not have any doughnuts. I am **choosing** to not go for the nachos. I use the word **choice**, because that's exactly what it is. I choose not to because I am choosing to lose weight, and have the body and health I always wanted.

I'm not going to lie to you, or pretend that it's easy. It is however, very doable. But as the person making the change, **you** have to find **your** voice. There is no more going along with the crowd. You are doing more. You are reaching higher, and to do so is going to take a serious commitment. You are committing to your health not what others think about you. They need to worry about them, and what they are choosing to do. You need to worry about you, and what you are choosing to do.

Jason: What were some of the reactions when the pounds started to come off?

Eli: People actually surprised me. I started losing weight, a lot of weight. It was obvious that my body was changing. People closest to me had the most discouraging things to say. I can remember friends approaching me, saying things like, *"Eli, how much weight are you gonna lose? Wow! Eli, aren't you overdoing it at the gym? You are so gung ho. Eli, are you becoming anorexic? You're no fun anymore. You don't look healthy. You are just obsessed! Eli, I hope you don't get too skinny."* And the classic, *"You think you're better than me don't you?"* I'm sure they all meant well, or at least, I would like to think they all meant well, but some of those comments were difficult to overcome. This road I am on, this road **WE** are traveling can be a lonely one at times, and that is why we have put so much focus on personal discipline. It's going to take strength to shake off those comments. It's going to take discipline to set goals, and believe in yourself enough to push past people's petty opinions. Do not expect the world to change for you, just because you are changing yourself. It won't.

Jason: My toughest critics ended up being my biggest supporters. What about you?

Eli: Exactly! That is exactly what I experienced. The guys telling me I couldn't make it, and teasing me when I was heading out to exercise were the same ones who came to me once the weight was all gone to ask me how to improve **their** workout, or what protein shakes **they** should drink. They changed so dramatically that I cannot leave them out of the book.

Those people trying to discourage you are only speaking to themselves. Their own fears are triggered, and they are trying to project those fears, doubts, and concerns on to you. Don't accept it. Stand up for yourself and feel stronger than ever before. Don't think. **Know** that you are on the right track. If you have set your goals with your doctor or health care provider, then who cares what anyone else thinks about it? It's not their problem and it's none of their business.

For those of you in relationships, it is very important that you remember a few things. You may have started your journey expecting your partner, spouse, or mate to fully support you. They may or they may not. People are all in different places in life, and you never know if your success is going be a benefit or a threat to your partner. Try not to judge them. You don't want to be judged, so show them the same courtesy. You are going on this journey because **YOU** want to. You aren't doing it for them. You don't know how they feel inside about themselves. So go easy on them. Measure your own success. Be thankful that they are willing, to go through your weight loss journey with you. You have agreed to go after your goals of health and fitness. They loved you before you even started this process. Remember that. Don't ever lose sight of the people who love you just the way you were. You have begun a process of transformation. You are going to grow stronger, more confident, more discipline and attract all kinds of new attention. Support your loved ones as they supported you throughout your transformation.

Jason: Since we started working on this project together, more and more people are asking me questions about your approach. Many of them want to know how a person can get over the fear or embarrassment of going out of the house to exercise in public.

Eli: That's actually pretty easy to explain. I bet the people asking were never afraid or embarrassed to order a double cheeseburger, pizza or a half-gallon of ice cream? They did not get to the point where I was by being shy about eating. I ate. Trust me. I ate plenty. Now that it's time to put the ice cream spoon down and pick some walking shoes up, there is no reason to be shy. Do you really believe that the sidewalk outside is just as much yours as anyone else's?

I used to believe that everyone driving by looked at me and said terrible things about me while I shuffled down the sidewalk. My shins hurt so bad I didn't think I could finish my 15 minutes of walking. I believed in my heart that the entire neighborhood was talking about me and joking about what I looked like trying to get in shape. But I believed in my commitment and pushed past my fears of judgment. I pushed. Now, after all that I've been through, I can tell you that the people driving by had their own lives to worry about. Many of them had health issues. Maybe, just maybe, by looking at me putting all that I had into my commitment and making my way down the sidewalk, I might've sparked some hope in them. They may, in turn, inspire someone else.

Jason: We will get in depth into that in the next chapter.

Eli: I understand, but at the same time I cannot stress enough how important it is to block out people's comments. You cannot afford to worry about what someone else is saying or thinking about your journey. It is **YOURS,** not theirs. When you are out there on your walk, imagine that everyone driving or walking by is saying: *"Wow! That guy is really making a change. Wow! She is getting her life back. What about me? What about* *my life? Will I ever get my fire back to get back in shape? What happened to me? I used to look good."* Chances are they're saying those kinds of things and more. In the rare case that a jerk makes a comment that hurts your feelings, feel sorry for him or her. One day, they may see you again and beg for your secret. Allow them to be ignorant. They have earned it.

Your journey and your personal commitment put you in the champion's circle. You have already begun your transformation. You have already proven that you care enough to read this far. You have that inner strength it takes to come this far. Go forward in happiness, knowing that you are finally making a new path for the good of you.

Jason: I have taken a lot of fire in my time. As a writer putting my own stories into the public domain, I have heard it all. People can be tough. Life can get a bit hard at times, but I have found through vision, determination, and commitment, I can do anything I set my mind to. Allow the negative people in your life to have a new role model. That's YOU!! Why not be the person they come to for advice? You will have the ability to tell them how you began to believe in yourself again and they can too.

"Fame is hollow. It amplifies what is there. If there is any self-doubt, or hatred, or lack of ability to connect with people, fame will magnify it."

Alanis Morissette

Chapter Sixteen: The Price of Success

Eli: You're on your way to the new you. It's important to fully understand what to expect. It's not all about exercise and dietary changes. Those things will help create a healthier, thinner you, but they cannot prepare you for the way the world may react to your success. Most of us have become experts at not being seen. We spend countless amounts of energy hiding in plain sight, blending in or going unnoticed. Our weight has heightened our self-consciousness and our fears about others looking at us.

I know that, on my journey, this was one of the hardest concepts to get used to. Years after the weight loss, I still looked at myself as a *big guy*. 110 pounds were physically gone, but those pounds were where I left them mentally...on my body. It took a great deal of time to get used to the fact that I was thin. But no matter how I looked at myself, no matter what I still thought of myself, the world saw me differently. The attention was a bit overwhelming at first. When I say *at first,* I mean for the first several years. This realization is critical for many.

You have to prepare yourselves to be seen! People are going to look at you. People are going to come up to you, and tell you that you look great. They are going to ask you how you did it. They will come to you for advice. Be ready. Try to tell yourself that these people are now looking to you for inspiration. They are not coming up to you to insult you, or tease you, or to judge you. Do your best to be gracious about it. It may be a bit disconcerting if you are a shy personality. Try your best to remain unafraid. You have worked very hard to lose the weight and get in shape; a little praise might be good for you.

Imagine for a minute that you didn't work on your body and health. Imagine that you designed a home. You spent hours and hours designing every square inch of that home and the surrounding property. When your home was finished, you held an 'open house.' People came from near and far to appraise your work. They told you how much they love the architecture, the interior decor and the landscaping. Would you be angry with them for complimenting your work? Would you be overly shy if they said they loved your taste? Would you throw them out for asking why you didn't design a house sooner? OF COURSE NOT! Of course, you wouldn't be angry with them. Yes, it might be hard being bombarded by compliments, but you would take them and feel appreciated for your efforts.
Why should it be any different with your body?

To the females, who have made it this far in my **One-Step-at-a-Time** approach to weight loss, I have a special message for you. Remember! Remember! And remember once more! The world we live in can be a visual place. Guys are very visual. At times, you may find yourself getting more attention than you ever had in your life. Your new body will attract attention from all directions. Taking a humble approach proves to be very effective. You may hate all of the attention. You may love it. Everyone is different. However, try and avoid getting caught up in it. Other women may be jealous of your new body. Men, who would have never approached you before this process, may come up to you with unexpected compliments. It's all part of life. People are people, and they do what they do. You have control over only one person...YOU!! Use that control you have built to be as kind as possible. Try to get used to the idea that many of your past hurdles are not going to turn to you for advice. Use your heart to forgive them for the ignorance they showed you. Be the bigger person in spirit because you won't be able to be the bigger person in body anymore. Enjoy your work. Be proud of all that you have accomplished.

Jason: What you're saying is so true. In my line of work, I come across many famous people. I find it fascinating that these folks dedicated their early years to becoming stars. The musicians practiced, and practiced to become one of the greats. The actors trained, and auditioned for years just to get a shot at their big break. But when the hard work paid off, and they became famous, something changed. It changed them. They started to both loathe and crave their newfound fame. I mean, they worked their whole lives to be noticed, but once it happened, they had to spent great fortunes to hide from the attention. Security guards, sunglasses, tinted limos and exclusive parties, VIP areas, velvet ropes keeping 'us' away from 'them.' And for what? Wasn't it their purpose in the first place to become famous enough someone would notice?

Of course, losing weight and becoming healthy isn't the same thing as starring in this summer blockbuster movie, but the concept is the same. You will be noticed. You will have people approach you. Enjoy the many fruits of your labor. Eli and I are going to go over techniques you can employ to make the experience a bit more meaningful. But overall, just enjoy yourself. You earned it!!

All good things in life take time. You are a great thing in life and it's going to take a little time at each stage for you to get used to it all.

Eli: Forgive your co-workers if they don't say the right things to you. They are speaking from where they are at that moment. Maybe they are depressed. Maybe they are jealous. Who know? It doesn't matter. You can't change them. You can only change you. You can only prepare yourself to be gracious. Forgive family members for doubting you. They were just doubting themselves. Let it go. Get over yourself and get over them. Now they see the new you, and they are stunned. Let them be stunned. It's always hard to get fans in your own hometown! Forgive your spouse or partner. Your strength has most likely scared the crap out of them. Many people will take your success as a slap in the face. Why do they do this? I may never know. But they do, so forgive them. You have a new power. You have a new superpower; so be a good hero. Be a kind of superhero. Be gentle with other people's feelings. Be especially kind to the harsher critics of your past. They may just turn out to be your biggest supporters.

Close your eyes and imagine a true champion from the past. When you see this winner, whether in business, sports, education, or civil rights, ask yourself: What of their character? Did they go around bragging about how great they were? Did they rub their success in everyone's face? Did they carry on like jerks, or as sources of inspiration? Chances are they were humble. Chances are they gave credit to all who helped them in their journey. You have that same spirit of a champion in you. Allow it to come out. Nurture it. Encourage it. Be that great. Be that humble. Be that wonderful. You deserve it. You deserve to be the champion that you already are on the inside. It's there waiting for you to let out. You have already won the battles. Now it is time to win the war. What is the war? The war is you accepting your greatness, you embracing your journey of success.

Success is one of the hardest things in the world to handle. It sounds silly, right? Well, it's not silly at all. It's real, and it makes the strongest among us fall to their knees. How do you accept success? You accept it by doing one single thing: Pay it forward!!

"Remember, if you ever need a helping hand, it's at the end of your arm, as you get older, remember you have another hand: The first is to help yourself, the second is to help others."

Audrey Hepburn

Chapter Seventeen: Paying It Forward

Eli: You are now well on your way to a new and improved you. Yes, there will be roadblocks and hurdles along the way, but you are building the tools to deal with those situations. You have learned that everything you need is already inside you. The first key is finding it; the second is letting it out. People ask me all the time: *"Eli, I heard how you got the weight off, but how did you keep it off for so long."* The answer is so simple most people don't hear it or don't believe it when they do hear it. It's all about **Paying it Forward.**

If I have something in life that only benefits me, I have a very limited view of what I am doing. However, when I include others in my journey, I expand my base and make myself much more stable. My view becomes broad, and my vision extended. By allowing myself to be a tool and resource for others, I give myself and my journey a much deeper meaning. I am now an instrument of change. Around the globe, I am a positive force for weight loss and fitness. This happened by making one simple decision: **To Share.** By sharing my experiences with others, I have made myself a conduit. I transport information from my experiences, as well as experiences I have gathered from other people, to people in need.

Jason: How do you find a person in need of the information?

ELI: I don't. They tend to find me. I don't believe in preaching to ears that are not open. I don't believe in approaching people, who don't think they need the information I have. No. That would be rude, and may do more harm to them than good. I allow people to approach me with questions. When they do approach me, I am more than happy to share what I know. We are both better for it. They get to learn that they are not alone, and what they want to do is not only possible, but doable. I walk away feeling better about myself because I helped another person. Because I feel better about myself, it tends to make me want to make better decisions. Making better decisions has become a habit for me. I love the positive energy that comes with it, so I repeat it as often as possible. For the person getting encouragement from me, the information they receive begins to restore their hope. Their newly-restored hope allows them to give the system a go. The results from their efforts make them believe in themselves a bit more and they try more. The more they try the better the results. The better the results, the better they feel about themselves. The better they feel about themselves, the more good they want to do. And so on. This cycle has no end. There is no finish line in doing good for other people. It just continues and expands.

Jason: It's been said that misery loves company. I believe the opposite is true, as well. Success loves success. Successful people are normally surrounded by other successful people. You are a success. There are people around you waiting and wanting to become successful, as well. When you communicate with them with like-minded goals, you are strengthening their resolve, as well as, your own.

Have you ever noticed how movie stars and famous musicians you love always seem to be wrapped up in one form of charity or another? What about the current generation of billionaires? Bill Gates, Warren Buffett, and Peter Lewis give away millions and millions of dollars. Why? They are trying to make the world a better place. They are using their gifts to gift to someone else. They are paying it forward and so can you.

You have taken upon yourself the noble task of improvement. Who better than you to encourage someone else? Who knows the struggles better than you do? Who can relate to the day-to-day hurdles people face when trying to improve their lives? YOU! YOU are the best thing going. Spread your gifts and they will return to you tenfold. The joy you receive will empower you to do more, give more, and be more than you every have in the past. GIVE.

Eli: There is another great benefit to paying it forward. It keeps you focused on the goal of getting and staying healthy. When you immerse yourself in your new lifestyle, it keeps your mind trained on that goal. When you know that others are depending on you to give advice the next morning, you will be less likely to slip up the night before and down that ice cream and soda. People are counting on you to take the walk in front of them. You are transforming yourself into a leader.

People ask me if I feel pressure now that I'm in shape and have people coming to me for advice. I always answer the same: NO! It isn't pressure. It's praise. It isn't a negative; it's a major positive. People can be shy. People can carry a lot of self-doubt. How wonderful it feels to know that I can help those people find their personal power. What an amazing gift I have been given to help others. I take it very seriously. When I am approached, for all I know, this person asking for advice might be too shy to ask anyone else but me. What if I give them a bunch of attitude, and they decide to never ask anyone again? How can that serve me? How can that help me grow stronger? You have read the stories of Rick and Jennifer. Those stories and many more stories like theirs inspire me to do more, reach higher, and tell more people my story. That has become my passion.

I was doing a promotional event when I was approached by a middle-aged man with a leg brace. I could easily tell he was not the type of guy to go around telling people about his problems. I asked him what he was struggling with. He told me he had recently suffered a stroke and didn't know the best way to deal with his new condition. I told him about my panic attacks, and how convinced I used to be that I was having a heart attack or a stroke almost all the time. I explained that my old weight and the two packs of cigarettes I smoked daily were leading me headfirst into a heart attack or stroke. I mentioned my three kids and proclaimed that I wanted to live to see them grow up. It struck a chord in him right away. He had two children. They were nearby, and when I saw him look at them, I could see the thought come over him. He turned to me and asked for my help. What more could I ask for as a reminder of just how important my role is? This man was asking me to help him live long enough to watch his children grow up. It once again reaffirmed that I am on the right track and I have been given a special and wonderful gift, a gift to **SHARE**!

Jason: One of the main reasons I write books is to pass on the experiences I have had in life, to help people not make the mistakes I have made in the past. However, I also write a lot about the successful moments in my life, and the lives of others. Countless times, I have been approached by people wanting to share their story with me. I listen intently. I know they are telling me things about their lives they may have never told another human being. It's important that I listen. It's important that I encourage them to be bold, and to own their thoughts and feelings. I know it's going to help them to be heard. I know it's going to allow them to accept themselves better, to know that they are not alone, or weird or crazy. So I listen. If I have any advice for them in the end, I will give it. If I don't, I will simply thank them for sharing. Either way, I am going to say something to them, and I am going to SHOW them that they matter and that their story needs to be heard...even if it's to be heard by me alone. I always encourage. I try to remember to never judge. I try to remember myself at my lowest point in life, and use that as a measuring stick against anyone else and what they may be going through. This allows me to be humble because I am reminded of the mistakes I have made. Actually, in most cases, the mistakes I have made were much worse than theirs. So I can relate. Relating is one of the human conditions that make us unique. Be unique. Enjoy it. Be it. It is exactly what makes you **YOU!**

Eli: We can learn a lot about ourselves by how we give to others. Are you a cheerful giver? Are you a bitter giver? How does it make you feel to help someone else? Answering those questions can tell you where you are, or where you come from. Giving is one of our greatest traits. If I hide all my secrets and never lift a finger to help another, what does that say about me? I don't want to be that person. Making others feel good brings me joy, encouragement, peace, humility, and understanding. It is what I do, and now it is who I am. I can finally say that I like who I am. I am who I want to be, and I want you to feel just as good about yourself as I do about me. Am I perfect? Not even close. But I am doing all that I can to be the kind of person I always wanted to be. That is the best I can do. And that is all that I ever asked for.

Thank you for spending the time with me through this book. You are welcome to stay in contact with me through my Facebook page:
https://www.facebook.com/FatBoyFitMan
Or on my website: www.fatboyfitman.com
I am excited for you to experience your journey. You are in good company. I believe in you. Now it's your turn to believe in you. This journey maybe the greatest gift you have ever given yourself. It is the gift that will get the weight off and keep the weight off. All you have to do is DO!! I will be there to see you through.

"Best advice that I ever got is to do whatever it takes to make myself happy, so that I'll be able to make others happy. If I'm not happy, I can't make other people happy."

Flavor Flav

Chapter Eighteen: In Review

Eli: I know there are a rare few, who have read this far in the book and still haven't decided to take the plunge into a new, fit, disciplined you. You are still waiting for a magic phrase, or special potion that is going to instantly transform you into a totally new person. Please let me know when you find it. All of us would become your customers overnight.

The truth is that there is no magical potion that will give you the power to achieve your dreams. There is hard work. There is dedication. There is humility. There is desire, and there is passion. Some of you are still waiting. You are still asking yourselves: *"Is Eli really talking to me?"* The answer is very simple: YES! YES! I am talking to you. In fact, I've been talking to you throughout this book! You are the reason I wrote the book in the first place. The people who get it right away are already off and doing the steps. This isn't for them. This is for you! I would assume you are still trying to figure out how to start, or if I even know what I'm talking about. I can understand you more than any other client I have. You have taken chances and exposed your hopes and dreams to a million different programs. They may have been all based on internal factors. My program is a bit different. My **One-Step-at-a-Time** Story of Success is based on decisions I made within myself. I rebuilt Eli from the inside out. By doing, I conditioned my mind and my body to think, act and feel dramatically different.

I am here for you. I have put down on paper what worked for me. It's really simple. You have to learn how to build discipline inside you. In addition, you have to make choices for yourself, to replace your bad food habits **One Step at a Time.** You are empowering yourself to start a form of exercise. You are going to do the exercise every day. You are going to be disciplined in the amount of time you exercise every day. If you say five minutes every day for a week, you do five minutes every day. You do not do two minutes or ten minutes. You do five. You are building discipline in yourself by doing so.

Jason: Remember the examples provided of others who have blazed a trail ahead of you. Thrive from their successes. The book is a tool to cover some of the most basic ideas in losing weight and getting healthy. What you eat and how much you exercise says so much about you. The idea is giving the power back to you. Getting you to take control of YOU is the point.

You might move to a new city. You may go through a promotion, or you might get fired. You never know. What you do know is that you can take control over your weight and your energy level. You can, in a sense, get your life back. We can't guarantee that you will never get sick for the rest of your life. However, you can take control and improve your body. Eli did it. Rick did it. Jennifer did it. Even I'm giving it a shot. It does work. It allows you to start thinking about what you are doing. It allows you to start helping yourself win a few of the battles at the table. Very few great things I have ever done were easy. However, all of the hard things I have done were great. It feels good to work. It feels good to become aware.

Jason Wood

Eli: Skeptics, finish the next chapter and go right back to the beginning of the book and start over. I want you to read it again. This time I want you to start the process, and perhaps, not talk about the fact that you think you might/ may/someday/think about the possibility that you may try to start it. **Just get out there and start doing it!!!** Going back to the start will allow you to read through it and use it as a reminder.

You are the one who is going to make all the choices.
You are the one who is going to transform.
You will not be the first one of us. However, you will be the most welcomed among us. The end of the journey is not what makes you one of us. Starting the journey is what does. I am with you and I believe not only that you can do it, but that you have been waiting to do it.

Eli Sapharti

"It had long since come to my attention that people of accomplishment rarely sat back and let things happen to them. They went out and happened to things."

Leonardo da Vinci

Dear Jessica, Moshe & Shuy,

Let me start by saying that I love each one of you so very much! You are my main reason for living and the main reason I continue to want to make a difference in the world. I am writing this letter to you in order to express some things that perhaps I have not said to you personally.

First of all, I am incredibly proud of you as individuals. You each have special qualities and strengths, but there are two qualities that all 3 of you share in common and those are KINDNESS & COMPASSION. These are qualities I learned from Mima, your grandmother, and I hope I passed on to you.

But, I do owe each one of you a sincere and long overdue apology.

I am truly sorry for having been such a horrible example in relation to living a healthy life. **I REALLY, REALLY, REALLY AM SO SORRY!**

As a parent, I thought that providing for you financially, giving you love, affection and attention was enough. It is **NOT!**

Until not too long ago did I realize the damage I had caused you by leading the unhealthy life that I did.

I AM SORRY!

I was teaching you that it was ok to smoke cigarettes one after the other. I taught you that it was ok to eat ANYTHING at ANYTIME in ANY QUANTITY! It is **NOT!**

I AM SORRY!

I showed you that lying around, sleeping the weekends away and not doing any physical activity was ok. It is **NOT!**

I AM SORRY!

I showed you that taking medication, going to see doctors and ending up in emergency rooms for something that I could have control over was not "my fault". It **WAS!**

I AM SORRY!

Not only did I show you many of these things by way of example, but also allowed for many of these bad habits to become part of your lives.

I AM TRULY SORRY!

Unfortunately I cannot change the past and the damage that was already done. But something I CAN teach you is that we are each in charge of our own destinies and that although I was not the best example or role model for many or most of your developing years, I hope that I AM today! Just as I took control of my life at the age of 38 and realized that no matter what mistakes I made in the past, I could still and at anytime STOP making those same mistakes and take steps towards "fixing" what I had messed up. SO CAN YOU!

You are each so young, vibrant, full of life and able to

live a life full of wonderful health! I hope and pray that in the last 5 years I have been able to correct at least some of the damage I have caused you by being a better example of how we should care for our health, our bodies and ultimately our lives.

I receive so many emails, messages and phone calls from people thanking me for being their source of inspiration and for helping them change their lives. And although it is incredibly rewarding and it brings me joy, it will not completely fulfill me until the three most important people in my life are just as affected by me as these others.

Everything positive I have done and accomplished has been fueled by your love support and unconditional acceptance of me. Every goal, dream and vision I have yet to reach is fueled by the thought that the three most important & wonderful people in my life are looking to me and counting on me to succeed. For this, **I THANK YOU!**

Jessica, Moshe, Shuy, each one of you has what it takes to make a great life for yourself and each one of you has the ability to pass that greatness to others, in turn making this a better world. You truly can accomplish **ANYTHING** you are passionate about. No matter how overwhelming it may seem at first, just remember to break down the seemingly impossible into possibilities and take it...

"One Step at a Time!"

I love you!

Dad

From Fat Boy to Fit Man

www.kantanoose.com